Colour Aids

Obstetrics

David James MA MD MRCOG DCH

Consultant Senior Lecturer in Obstetrics,
University Department of Obstetrics,
Bristol Maternity Hospital,
Bristol, UK

Mary Pillai MRCP (UK) MRCOG DCH

Research Fellow in Feto-maternal Medicine,
University Department of Obstetrics,
Bristol Maternity Hospital,
Bristol, UK

Churchill Livingstone

EDINBURGH LONDON MELBOURNE AND NEW YORK 1990

Acknowledgements

We are grateful to the following for providing some of the illustrations for this book: Professor G.M. Stirrat, Dr B. Spiedel, Mr P. Savage, Dr P. Burton, Dr R. Slade, Dr D. Warnock, Dr A. Jeffcote, Dr N. Hunter, Dr J. Haworth, Dr H. Andrews and Dr J. Pardey. We are especially indebted to Mr N. Bowyer, of the Department of Medical Illustration, Southmead Hospital, Bristol, for his advice and practical help in the preparation of illustrations.

Contents

Early Pregnancy (1)

Fertilization and implantation

Fertilization of the ovum by sperm occurs in the outer third of the Fallopian tube. The division of the blastocyst reaches a 4-cell stage (Fig. 1) after 36–48 hours. The blastocyst arrives in the uterus at 72–96 hours (16 cells) and remains free in the uterine cavity for 4–5 days. Implantation occurs 6–9 days after fertilization. Primitive chorionic villi develop at 13–15 days. The gestational sac is visible on ultrasound (U/S) by 5–6 weeks (Fig. 2).

Early diagnosis of pregnancy

For clinical features of pregnancy, see pp. 5–8. Human chorionic gonadotrophin (hCG) is a glycoprotein hormone secreted by the trophoblastic cells of the placenta. It is present in the urine of pregnant women and is a useful marker for diagnosing pregnancy. Initially agglutination inhibition assays were used, followed by radioimmunoassays. More recently, the development of monoclonal antibodies to hCG have improved the sensitivity so that a simple, quick kit test (Fig. 3) can now reliably detect as little as 50 mU/ml of hCG—the level found approximately 10 days after conception. *The expected date of delivery* (EDD) is 7 days and 9 months after the first day of the last normal menstrual period.

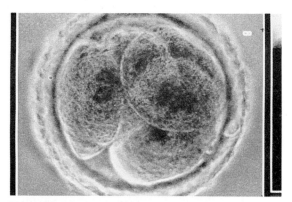

Fig. 1 Blastocyst: 4-cell stage.

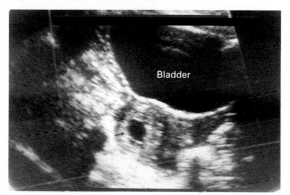

Bladder

Fig. 2 U/S of gestational sac (5–6 weeks) (arrowed).

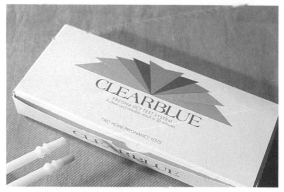

Fig. 3 Pregnancy test (blue = positive).

Early Pregnancy (2)

Fetal growth and development

The first 3 months of pregnancy (trimester) represent a period of rapid fetal growth and development.

Fetal growth
The pattern of fetal growth shows little variability in the first half of pregnancy when genetic control is dominant. The influence of non-genetic factors gives rise to greater variability in later pregnancy. Growth in the first half of pregnancy can be recorded by ultrasound (Figs. 4 and 5) using the crown-rump length (CRL) (8–14 weeks) and/or biparietal diameter (BPD) (from 12 weeks).

Menstrual age (weeks)	CRL (mm)	BPD (mm)	Fetal wt (g)
8 (Fig. 4)	15	—	—
10	33	—	—
12 (Fig. 5)	58	18	14
14 (Fig. 6)	80	26	36
16	—	35	97

Fetal development
The organ systems are formed during the first trimester—the period of embryogenesis/organogenesis.

Organ system	Approximate gestational age at formation (weeks)
Limbs	6–10
Heart	5–10
Central nervous system	5–11
Eye	6–7
Ear	9–10

Pathology

Fetal growth and development may be seriously affected by a variety of factors in the first trimester including maternal diabetes (p. 55), infections (p. 15), drugs (p. 59) and genetic abnormalities (p. 25).

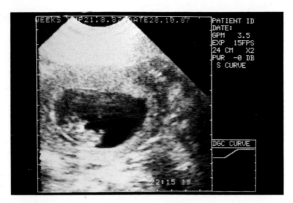

Fig. 4 U/S of 8-week fetus.

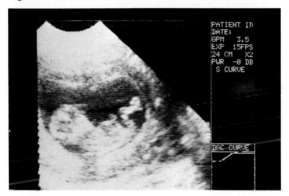

Fig. 5 U/S of 12-week fetus.

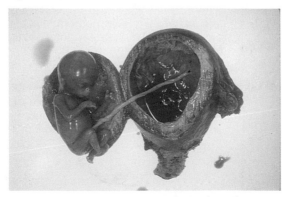

Fig. 6 14-week pregnancy hysterectomy specimen.

2 | Normal Pregnancy and Care (1)

Aims of care

Pregnancy in most cases will be a normal event with low risk of harm to mother or baby. For a few, however, there is a greater risk of adverse outcome for mother and/or baby. The aims of antenatal care are:
1. To provide appropriate surveillance to assess the degree of risk of harm to mother and/or baby.
2. a. For those at low risk with no significant problems in normal pregnancies, to provide advice, education and support.
   b. For those at some risk of maternal/fetal harm, to provide additional care which will prevent, minimize or treat the problems.

History

At the first visit, the following data are recorded: maternal age, marital status, menstrual, medical and surgical, obstetric, family and social histories and details of any problems. Alcohol and smoking habits are also documented. At subsequent visits any new problems are noted, together with maternal perception of fetal movements.

Symptoms

Amenorrhoea and tiredness are common early symptoms. Most organ systems may be affected in pregnancy—gastrointestinal (nausea, vomiting, oesophagitis, constipation, gum hypertrophy (Fig. 7)), urogenital (frequency), breasts (tingling, enlargement) (Fig. 8), skin (pigmentation) (Fig. 9), cardiorespiratory (palpitations, breathlessness).

Advice and support

The woman with a normal pregnancy is given advice and education during her pregnancy on diet and breastfeeding. She is strongly advised not to smoke or drink alcohol.

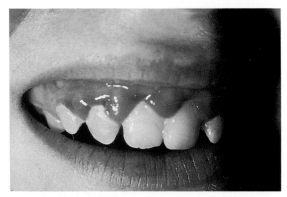

Fig. 7 Gum hypertrophy.

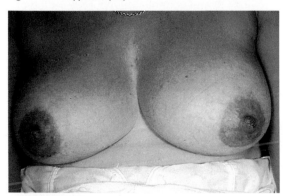

Fig. 8 Breast changes.

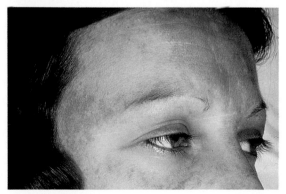

Fig. 9 Chloasma.

Examination

At the first visit a full general examination is undertaken. At all visits weight, blood pressure (see p. 51), uterine size, fetal number, lie and presentation are recorded. In later pregnancy the engagement of the fetal head is noted and the fetal heart is auscultated.

Signs

Early signs of pregnancy include changes in the breasts (enlargement, pigmentation, venous engorgement, and Montgomery's tubercles) (Fig. 8) and genitalia (bluish colouration of vaginal skin and cervix, softening and enlargement of uterus). Other signs include: gum hypertrophy (Fig. 7), chloasma (Fig. 9), striae gravidarum (Fig. 10), linea nigra, umbilical pigmentation and eversion (Fig. 11), lymphadenopathy, thyroid enlargement (a soft systolic murmur may be physiological, oedema is found in 60% of normal pregnancies) and varicose veins (Fig. 12).

Investigations

At the first visit, urinalysis is undertaken (glucose, protein, ketones) and a midstream sample of urine (MSU) is sent for culture. Blood is taken for full blood count and film, ABO and rhesus grouping, antibody screening, rubella antibody status and serological test for syphillis. Screening for fetal neural tube defect may be performed by maternal serum alpha-feto-protein (AFP) estimation at 16 weeks. At subsequent visits, urinalysis is always undertaken and, for example, MSU at 30 weeks, full blood count at 26 and 34 weeks, rhesus antibodies in rhesus-negative mothers at 26 and 34 weeks.

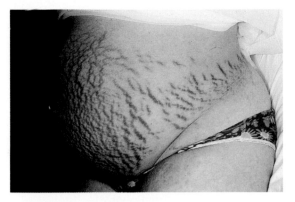

Fig. 10 Striae gravidarum.

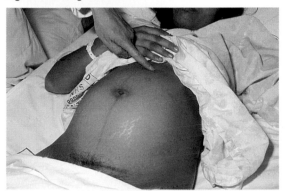

Fig. 11 Linea nigra and umbilical pigmentation and eversion.

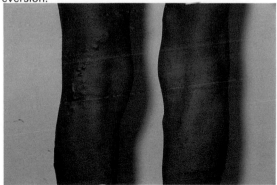

Fig. 12 Varicose veins.

Complications of Early Pregnancy (1)

Abortion

Definition

'Expulsion of the products of conception before the 28th week of pregnancy where the fetus shows no signs of life after delivery.' Most abortions occur in the first 12 weeks.

Terminology

Threatened abortion: uterine bleeding but the pregnancy continues.
Inevitable abortion: bleeding, uterine contractions (pain), the cervix dilates and the products of conception are expelled (Fig. 13). It is *complete* when all the products have been expelled, and *incomplete* when not all the products of conception have been expelled.
Missed abortion: the fetus dies but the products of conception are retained in the uterus.
Septic abortion: abortion caused by or associated with infection.
Blighted ovum: an empty gestational sac with collapsed outline and no fetal node (Fig. 14).

Aetiology

Fetal abnormalities (especially chromosomal) are the commonest causes. Others include infection, congenital uterine anomalies, fibroids, uterine scars, cervical incompetence.

Clinical features

Amenorrhoea, colicky pain/ache (40%), bleeding (98%), shock (5%), cervical dilatation and passage of products (15%).

Complications

Anaemia, shock, infection, disseminated intravascular coagulation, depression/grief.

Management

Complete and inevitable abortions may require no more than analgesia. Incomplete and missed abortions require uterine curettage. Blood transfusion may be required. Psychological support is important.

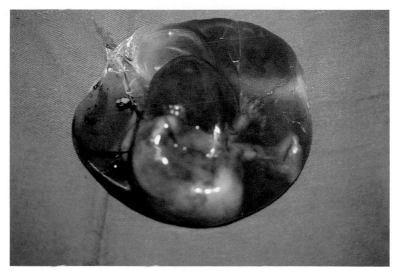

Fig. 13 Aborted abnormal fetus and placenta (10 weeks).

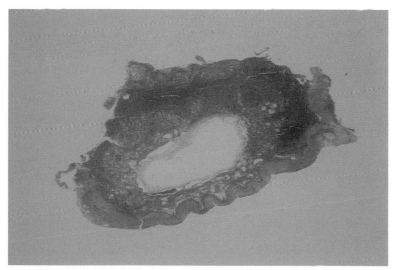

Fig. 14 Histological section of blighted ovum (empty gestation sac).

3 | Complications of Early Pregnancy (2)

Ectopic pregnancy

Definition and incidence

'Implantation of a pregnancy in a site other than the normal uterodecidual area'. Occurs in 1 in 150 live births. The commonest site is the Fallopian tube (Figs. 15 and 16) but others include the ovary (Fig. 17) and abdominal cavity. It is more commonly found in women with an intrauterine contraceptive device (Fig. 15), a previous ectopic pregnancy, or a history of pelvic infection or tubal surgery.

Clinical features

The pregnancy distending the Fallopian tube produces lower abdominal pain on one side. There may be some dark red vaginal bleeding due to decidual breakdown. Clinical features of pregnancy and a positive pregnancy test are not always found. On examination, the uterus may be soft and slightly enlarged, with positive cervical excitation and tenderness often with a mass to one side of the uterus. Tube rupture (approximately 10% of cases) will produce sudden pain followed by shock and collapse. Shoulder tip pain can be experienced due to subdiaphragmatic irritation by intraperitoneal blood.

Management

Pregnancy test, laparoscopy, pelvic ultrasound (Fig. 15) and paracentesis may aid in the diagnosis. However, laparotomy and removal of the ectopic (usually by salpingectomy, with or without oophorectomy) is the definitive treatment. Transfusion of blood may be necessary.

Sequelae

There is an increased incidence of subfertility (50%) and about 10% suffer a further ectopic pregnancy in the contralateral tube.

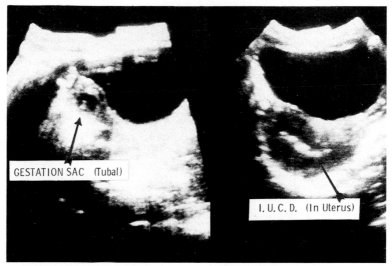

Fig. 15 U/S showing uterus with coil (right) and ectopic (left).

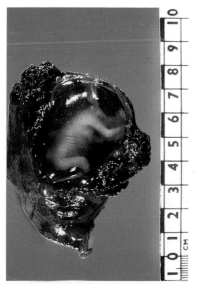

Fig. 16 Tubal ectopic pregnancy (opened).

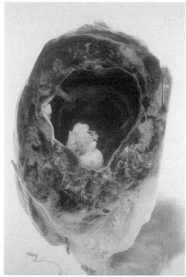

Fig. 17 Ovarian ectopic pregnancy.

Complications of Early Pregnancy (3)

Trophoblastic disease

Definition and incidence

'Neoplasia occurring in the placenta'. The incidence is 1:600 in the Far East but 1:2000 in the West. The villi become grossly hydropic with invasive properties and endocrine activity.

Types

The majority are benign (Fig. 20) (hydatidiform mole) although pseudomalignant, being capable of invading the myometrium and being carried in the blood. There are two types: complete (Fig. 19) and partial (Fig. 18). Very occasionally, a complete mole can become malignant (Fig. 21) (choriocarcinoma). A partial mole hardly ever becomes malignant but is always found in association with a triploid fetus.

Clinical features

Uterine bleeding, often after amenorrhoea and exaggerated features of pregnancy are features of trophoblastic disease. In 50% of cases the uterus is larger than expected from the duration of amenorrhoea; in 25% it is smaller. There is a higher incidence of pre-eclampsia. Features of thyrotoxicosis are occasionally present. Villi may be visible through the cervix.

Diagnosis

Diagnosis is often made at currettage for presumed incomplete abortion. The levels of hCG are greatly elevated and ultrasound reveals a 'snow-storm' picture.

Management

Initially the uterus is emptied by suction and curettage and subsequent monitoring is by urinary and/or blood beta-hCG levels. Levels which fail to fall or rise subsequently suggest incomplete evacuation, invasion, metastasis or malignant change and in these cases chemotherapy is undertaken. Hysterectomy is rarely indicated.

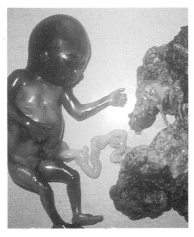

Fig. 18 Partial mole with triploid fetus.

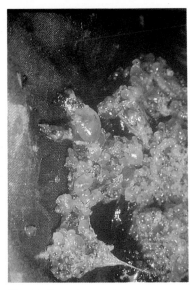

Fig. 19 Complete mole.

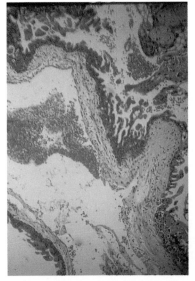

Fig. 20 Benign trophoblastic disease (hydatidiform mole).

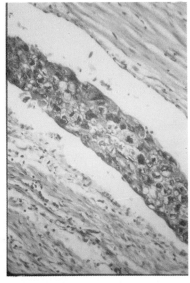

Fig. 21 Malignant trophoblastic disease (choriocarcinoma).

Rubella

Mother

Clinical
Exposure 2–3 weeks earlier, 3-day maculopapular rash, lymphadenopathy, fever, malaise, conjunctivitis and cough.

Laboratory
Elevated haemgglutination antibody, specific rubella IgM antibody (falls after 3 months), virus from throat.

Management
Avoid pregnant women.

Baby

Clinical
Significant permanent organ damage with maternal infection in 50% in the first month, 22% in the second month, 10% in the third month and 1% after four months. Eye problems, heart defects, microcephaly, mental retardation, thrombocytopenic purpura (Fig. 22), hepatosplenomegaly, small-for-dates.

Laboratory
Haemagglutination antibody elevation (beyond 3 months), specific rubella IgM antibody, virus from throat, urine and spinal fluid.

Management
Isolate (virus shed for 6–12 months), with careful assessment and follow-up.

Toxoplasmosis

Mother
Often asymptomatic, and there may be history of cat contact or raw meat ingestion. Diagnosis is by seroconversion, titre rise or placental histology (Fig. 24).

Baby
Clinical features include chorioretinitis, convulsions, hydrocephaly and intracranial calcification (Fig. 23), thrombocytopenic purpura, hepatosplenomegaly, jaundice, fever, pneumonitis and small for dates. Treatment is supportive.

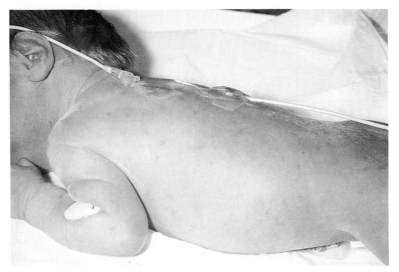

Fig. 22 Infant with congenital rubella.

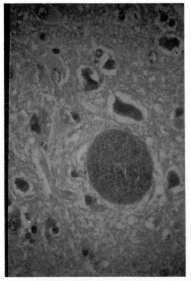

Fig. 23 Toxoplasmosis—fetal brain, microscopic appearance.

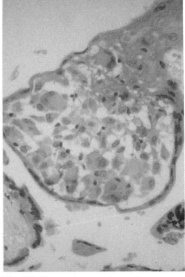

Fig. 24 Toxoplasmosis—placenta.

Congenital Infections (2)

Cytomegalovirus

Mother
Almost always asymptomatic. If cytomegalovirus
is suspected then isolation of the virus from cervix
urine is possible.

Baby
90% of cases are asymptomatic while severe fetal
infection results in perinatal death. The remainder
have thrombocytopenic purpura (Fig. 25), hepatosplenomegaly, chorioretinitis, microphthalmia,
nephritis (Fig. 26), microcephaly, deafness,
mental retardation, cerebral calcification and
small-for-dates. Diagnosis is by virus isolation.

Herpes simplex

Mother
Genital infection is sexually transmitted (see also
p. 57). Painful vesicles are found on the cervix,
vagina and external genitalia (Fig. 103). Primary
infection (multiple lesions and often lymphadenopathy) lasts for 1 week; recurrent infections
(fewer, less painful lesions) lasts for 3−4 days.
Diagnosis is clinical, cytological or by viral
culture. Acyclovir has been safe and successful
after the first trimester. Caesarean section is
considered if delivery is anticipated within 2
weeks of active genital herpes.

Baby
Infection (from vaginal delivery with active
herpes) can be disseminated (70%) (jaundice,
purpura, respiratory distress,
hepatosplenomegaly, encephalitis), localized
(15%) (lesions on face) or central nervous system
only (15%) (encephalitis).

Parvovirus

This virus can produce fetoplacental infection
with fetal death due to hydrops (Figs. 27 and 28).

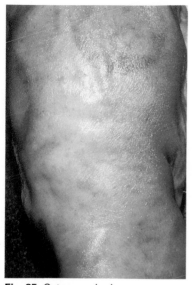

Fig. 25 Cytomegalovirus—cutaneous manifestations on trunk.

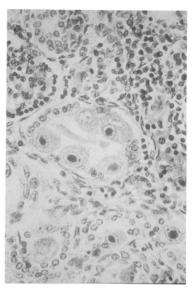

Fig. 26 Cytomegalovirus—kidney.

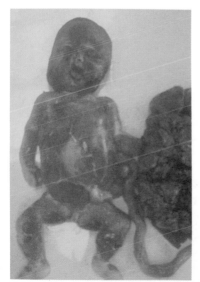

Fig. 27 Parvovirus—hydropic fetus and placenta.

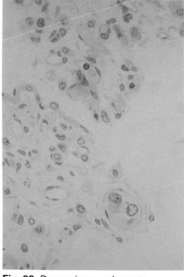

Fig. 28 Parvovirus—placenta.

Congenital Infections (3)

Listeriosis

Mother
Caused by *Listeria monocytogenes*, listeriosis is usually asymptomatic, occasionally producing a 'flu'-like illness. It very rarely presents as septicaemia.

Baby
Pregnancy may end in abortion or fetal death. In survivors there are two types.
1. *Early-onset:* diffuse septicaemia with cutaneous (Fig. 29), pulmonary, hepatic and neurological involvement (mortality 90%). The babies are small-for-dates.
2. *Late onset:* (possibly acquired after birth) meningitis with mental retardation and/or hydrocephalus (mortality 40%). Diagnosis is by isolation of the organism (Fig. 30); treatment is with ampicillin or erythromycin.

Syphillis

Mother
The risk of congenital syphillis varies with stage of maternal infection—50% with *primary* (chancre) and *secondary* (disseminated lymphadenopathy and rash); 40% with *latent* and 10% with *late* (gummas, neurological and cardiovascular). Diagnosis is by isolation of the organism (primary and secondary) and serological tests. Seropositive mothers are usually treated with penicillin irrespective of the risk to the fetus.

Baby
In severe congenital infection the placenta and fetus are hydropic and the fetus often still-born. Most are asymptomatic and may be seropositive or negative (recent infection). An uninfected newborn may be seropositive because of passive transfer. A few will manifest early congenital syphillis (Figs. 31 and 32) (rash, hepatosplenomegaly, lymphadenopathy, oedema). Treatment is with penicillin.

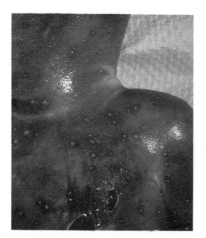

Fig. 29 Listeriosis—cutaneous manifestations.

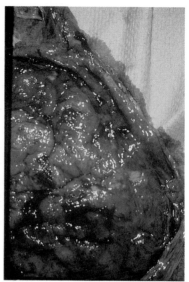

Fig. 30 Listeriosis—placenta.

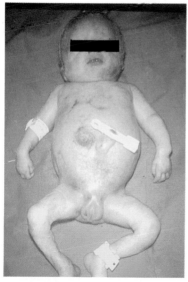

Fig. 31 Syphillis—fetus.

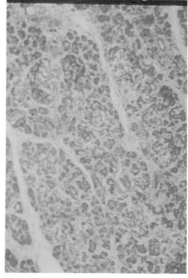

Fig. 32 Syphillis—pancreatic fibrosis.

5 | Prenatal Diagnosis (1)

General

Over the last 15 years dramatic advances have been made in prenatal diagnosis.
Obstetric procedures are performed under ultrasound control. Ultrasound is also the most important method in prenatal diagnosis (p. 29). The methods include chorion villus sampling (placental biopsy), amniocentesis, cordocentesis and fetal tissue biopsy. Such invasive procedures also allow fetal therapy to be undertaken, e.g. fetal blood transfusion for rhesus disease (p. 45) and in certain cases of urethral valves to insert a vesico-amniotic shunt.
Laboratory methods include chromosome analysis (karyotyping) (either directly or after fetal cell culture), DNA analysis, enzyme assay and measurement of haematological values.

Chorionic villus sampling (CVS)

The method used (usually in the first trimester) can be transcervical biopsy or aspiration (Figs. 33 and 34) or transabdominal aspiration, which is similar to amniocentesis (p. 23). The transabdominal approach can also be used after the first trimester. After chorionic villi have been confirmed at the bedside (Figs. 35 and 36) they may be used for chromosome analysis, DNA analysis (e.g. haemoglobinopathies, Duchenne muscular dystrophy) and enzymology (inborn errors of metabolism). Possible risks include abortion (2–6%), rupture of membranes, rhesus sensitization, infection and uterine trauma.

OBSTETRICS

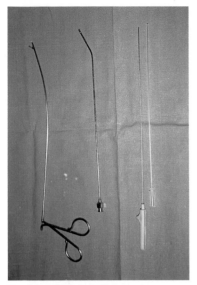

Fig. 33 CVS—transcervical instruments (aspiration or biopsy).

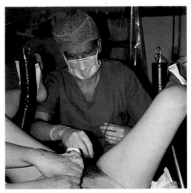

Fig. 34 CVS—transcervical biopsy under ultrasound guidance.

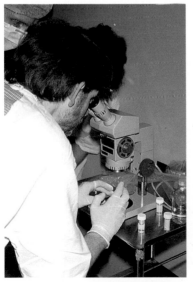

Fig. 35 CVS—bedside low-power identification of chorionic villi.

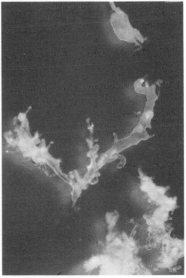

Fig. 36 CVS—low-power view of chorionic villi.

5 | Prenatal Diagnosis (2)

Amniocentesis

Procedure

Amniotic fluid is obtained by inserting a 20-gauge spinal needle (Fig. 37) into the amniotic cavity transabdominally under ultrasound guidance (Figs. 38, 39 and 40), after the first trimester (usually 16 weeks).

Indications

Chromosome analysis (for chromosomal abnormalities, fetal sexing in X-linked conditions), additional confirmation of neural tube defects (alpha-feto-protein and acetylcholinesterase), inborn errors of metabolism (enzymes, metabolites using cell or supernatant), DNA analysis (where there is a gene probe for a specific condition) and later in pregnancy for assessment of rhesus disease (p. 45).

Risks

Maternal: delay for result (3−4 weeks with karyotype), infection, haematoma and psychological problems.
Fetal/neonatal: abortion (about 0.5%), trauma, haemorrhage, preterm rupture of membranes, labour, rhesus sensitization, respiratory distress and postural deformities.

Cordocentesis and other techniques

The aspiration of fetal blood from the umbilical cord after 18 weeks is performed to diagnose inherited haemoglobin disorders, inborn errors of metabolism, karyotyping, fetal viral infection, rhesus disease, unexplained hydrops and fetal anaemia. Risks include abortion, trauma, blood loss, fetal death, preterm rupture of membranes and labour, and rhesus sensitization. Fetal skin and liver biopsy have been undertaken in the diagnosis of lethal conditions. Fetoscopy (direct visualization of the fetus) is now superceded by the above techniques.

OBSTETRICS

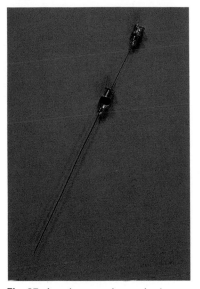

Fig. 37 Amniocentesis—spinal needle.

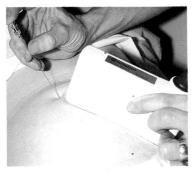

Fig. 38 Amniocentesis—insertion of needle under ultrasound guidance.

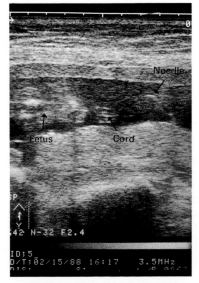

Fig. 39 Amniocentesis—ultrasound picture.

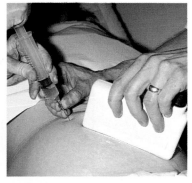

Fig. 40 Amniocentesis—aspiration of liquor.

6 | Chromosomal Abnormalities (1)

Down's syndrome (trisomy 21)

Incidence

Occurs in 1 in 600 live births, and shows increasing incidence with older mothers (1 in 2000 at age 25, 1 in 365 at 35, 1 in 100 at 40). Overall recurrence risk is 1%, (higher if there is a balanced translocation or if the mother is over 40 years of age).

Antenatal diagnosis

Offered to mothers aged 38 years or more. A low alpha-feto-protein may predict an increased risk in mothers aged 32–37.

Aetiology

Trisomy 21 in 94% of cases (Fig. 41), translocation in 3% and mosaicism in 3%.

Clinical features

Miscarriage/fetal death, small-for-dates, mongoloid facies, hypotonia, brachycephaly, single palmar creases, digit abnormalities, and often other congenital anomalies (e.g. heart) (Fig. 42). Mental retardation is common. Mean age of survival is 30–40 years.

Edward's syndrome (trisomy 18/E)

Incidence

Occurs in 1 in 3000 live births; as with Down's syndrome, increased risk with advancing maternal age. Recurrence risk is low.

Aetiology

Trisomy 18 (Fig. 43).

Clinical features

Miscarriage/fetal death, small-for-dates, severe mental retardation, hypoplastic lungs, flexion deformities, clenched fist with outer fingers overlapping the middle two, rocker-bottom feet, and craniofacial abnormalities (Fig. 44). Other congenital abnormalities are common (cardiac, urogenital). The majority die within a few months; less than 10% survive more than 1 year.

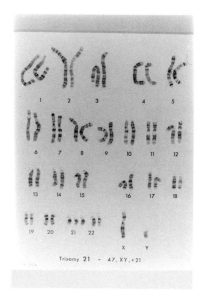

Fig. 41 Trisomy 21 karyotype.

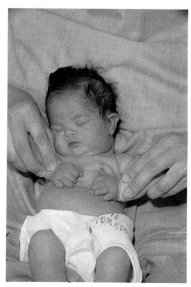

Fig. 42 Baby with Down's syndrome (trisomy 21).

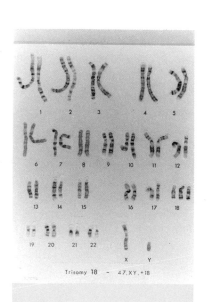

Fig. 43 Trisomy 18/E karyotype.

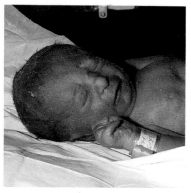

Fig. 44 Baby with Edward's syndrome (trisomy 18/E).

Chromosomal Abnormalities (2)

Patau's syndrome (trisomy 13/D)

Incidence

Uncommon with a low recurrence risk. Higher risk in older women.

Aetiology

Trisomy 13 (Fig. 45).

Clinical features

Patau's syndrome can present as miscarriage/fetal death, small-for-dates, midline defects of face, eyes and forebrain, cleft lip and palate (Fig. 46). Severe mental retardation, deafness, rocker-bottom feet, congenital heart defects, and cryptorchidism. Less than 20% survive the first year of life.

Turner's syndrome (45, XO)

Incidence

Occurs in 1 in 5000 live births; incidence is usually sporadic.

Aetiology

Single X chromosome (45, XO) (Fig. 47).

Clinical features

Turner's syndrome can present as miscarriage or fetal death often with a cystic hygroma or hydrops (Fig. 48). Common features include small-for-dates, phenotypically female infants with transient lymphoedema of limbs, neck webbing, broad chest with widely spaced nipples, low hairline and short neck, and cubitus valgus. In approximately 10%, coarctation of aorta and mild mental retardation occurs.

Prognosis

Short stature, failure of secondary sexual development usually corrected with cyclical oestrogen from adolescence. Normally infertile. Usually normal intelligence and life expectancy

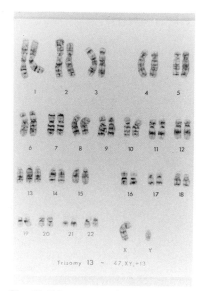

Fig. 45 Trisomy 13/D karyotype.

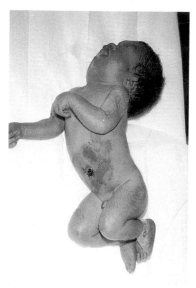

Fig. 46 Fetus with Patau's syndrome (trisomy 13/D).

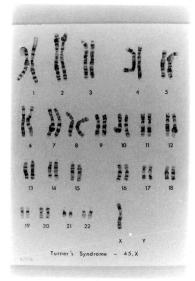

Fig. 47 45, XO karyotype.

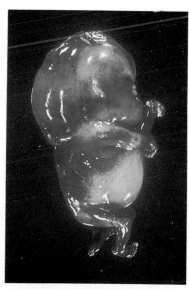

Fig. 48 Fetus with Turner's syndrome (45, XO).

7 | Obstetric Ultrasound

General

Approximately 70% of mothers in the UK have a routine scan in the first half of pregnancy and a further 15% have a scan later.

Principles

A variety of obstetric real-time diagnostic ultrasound machines are employed (Fig. 49). They all work on similar basic principles with a probe (Fig. 50) applied to the maternal abdomen using a film of gel (to ensure good contact). There are two types of probe: (i) a linear or curvilinear probe containing a series (about 40) of ultrasound transmitters and receivers; or (ii) a sector probe which has no more than three or four transmitters and receivers. The identification of structures in the ultrasound beam occurs by the same principle as sonar or radar. Diagnostic imaging uses a 1 us pulse of ultrasound (usually 3.5 mHz) followed by a 1 ms gap for detection of the returning sound wave. By sequencing the firing of the transmitters in rapid succession a real-time image is obtained (Figs. 51 and 52).

Applications

Determining fetal viability, diagnosing fetal abnormality, multiple pregnancy and trophoblastic disease. In the first half of pregnancy, it is used to assess gestational age, in the latter half of pregnancy, for determining placental site and fetal presentation, documenting fetal growth and behaviour, and measuring liquor volume. It is a mandatory adjunct for invasive procedures such as amniocentesis.

Safety

The evidence supports the view that ultrasound is safe for mother, baby and operator.

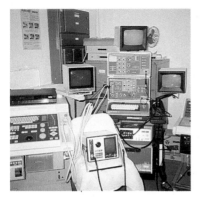

Fig. 49 Real-time ultrasound machines.

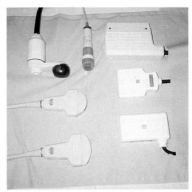

Fig. 50 Ultrasound probes.

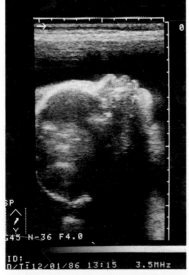

Fig. 51 Linear array scanner picture.

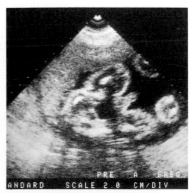

Fig. 52 Sector scanner picture.

Congenital Abnormalities (1)

Neural tube defects (NTD)

Types

Spina bifida (meningomyelocele, meningocele), anencephaly, encephalocele.

Incidence

Overall occurrence is 1 in 300 but displays geographical variation.

Aetiology and prevention

Unknown but nutritional deficiency possible. Risk of recurrence (1 in 20) may be reduced if the mother takes folate with or without multivitamins from at least 1 month preconception and through the first trimester.

Antenatal diagnosis

Many areas offer mothers serum alpha-feto-protein screening at 16–18 weeks. A value below 2.3–2.5 times the population median indicates a low risk of NTD. A raised value makes NTD more likely but other causes include fetal abdominal wall defects, multiple pregnancy, incorrect gestational age and bleeding in pregnancy. When the alpha-feto-protein value is raised, a detailed scan is undertaken (Fig. 53). If then the diagnosis is still uncertain an amniocentesis is performed—a raised amniotic fluid alpha-feto-protein and the presence of acetylcholinesterase would be diagnostic of NTD.

Spina bifida
A fluid-filled sac often containing neural tissue and an underlying defect of the spinal arch. 94% are lumbosacral. The degree of handicap varies and can include lower limb paralysis, urinary and faecal incontinence, limb deformities, hip dislocations, urinary infections, hydrocephalus (70%) (Fig. 54).

Encephalocele
Herniation of the meninges and brain through the skull (usually occipital).

Anencephaly
Absence of the forebrain and skull vault, facial distortion (Figs. 55 and 56). Other abnormalities are common. Incompatible with life.

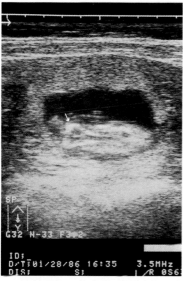

Fig. 53 U/S at 15 weeks; splaying of lower lumbar spine arrowed.

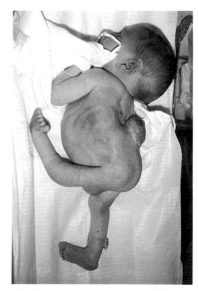

Fig. 54 Newborn with spina bifida.

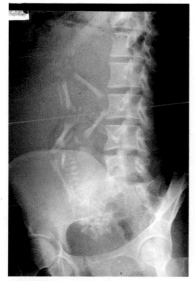

Fig. 55 X-ray of fetus in utero with anencephaly (no vault bones).

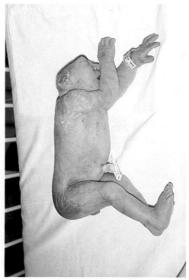

Fig. 56 Anencephalic baby.

Hydrocephalus

Definition

Excessive accumulation of intraventricular cerebrospinal fluid (Figs. 57 and 58).

Aetiology

May be isolated, secondary to aqueduct stenosis or intraventricular haemorrhage. Most common associated abnormality is a NTD (and the Arnold Chiari malformation).

Antenatal diagnosis

The alpha-feto-protein is normal with a closed NTD. Diagnosis is made with ultrasound (increased ventriculohemispheric ratio) (Figs. 59 and 60).

Prognosis

This varies. Babies with isolated defects may be born with accelerating rate of growth of the skull and a shunt may be required; even then the child may be irreversibly handicapped. Conversely, even if the hydrocephalus is not progressing at birth the baby may be handicapped, although in a few cases may develop normally.
Intra-uterine surgical procedures are of no benefit. If there is an underlying major abnormality (such as NTD), predicting the prognosis is relatively easier.

Microcephaly

Definition and antenatal diagnosis

This requires ultrasonic demonstration of fetal head circumference below third centile for age and gestation which is disproportionately smaller than abdominal circumference and femur length.

Aetiology

Often unknown, but may be familial. Pathological causes include congenital viral infections and certain congenital abnormalities (e.g. Down's syndrome). The prognosis depends on the cause.

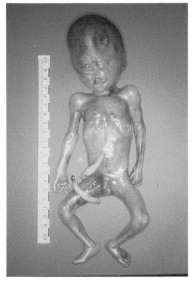

Fig. 57 Fetus with hydrocephalus.

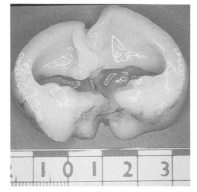

Fig. 58 Macroscopic appearance of brain section.

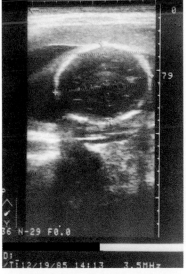

Fig. 59 Normal U/S appearance of fetal head.

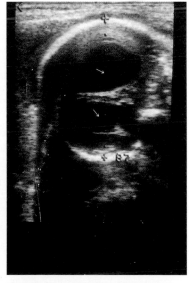

Fig. 60 U/S of fetal head showing dilated ventricles. (arrowed)

Abdominal wall defects

Gastroschisis and exomphalos

Pathology

Uncommon conditions, with unknown aetiologies. Failure of rotation and re-entry of gut into abdominal cavity during fetal development.

Features

Associated with elevated maternal serum alpha-feto-protein levels. Diagnosed by ultrasound.
Gastroschisis (Figs. 61 and 62): defect of the abdominal wall separate from the insertion of the umbilicus. The abdominal viscera herniate, usually the peritoneal covering is lost (Figs. 61 and 62). Usually an isolated defect.
Exomphalos (Fig. 63): herniation of the abdominal viscera through a defect at the umbilicus. Usually peritoneal covering is preserved and umbilical cord is inserted at the apex of the sac. Other congenital abnormalities are common (cardiac, bowel and chromosomal).

Management

Depends on associated anomalies. If not lethal, surgical closure is undertaken as soon as possible after birth. This may be as a two-stage procedure, with the abdominal contents being enclosed in a temporary artificial sac initially. Mode of delivery does not influence the prognosis.

Prune belly syndrome (Fig. 64)

Incidence

Uncommon, with only sporadic occurrence.

Features

Deficient abdominal wall musculature, giving a rugose prune-belly appearance. Undescended testes and renal anomalies associated.

Management

Depends on the renal anomalies. If not lethal, abdominal wall is reconstructed in infancy.

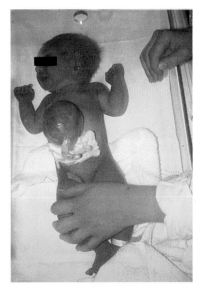

Fig. 61 U/S scan of fetal abdomen (gastroschisis and cord separately arrowed).

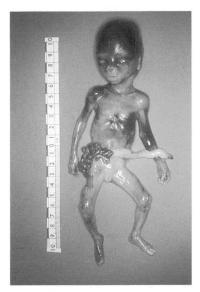

Fig. 62 Gastroschisis.

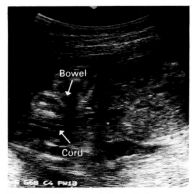

Fig. 63 Exomphalos.

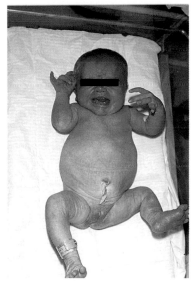

Fig. 64 Prune belly syndrome.

Renal tract anomalies

Potter's syndrome (Fig. 65)

Incidence

Occurs in 1 in 3000 live births.

Aetiology

The syndrome (Fig. 65) is produced by any condition resulting in oligohydramnios. Thus renal agenesis (the cause of the original description of Potter's syndrome), dysplastic kidneys (Fig. 67), polycystic kidneys (Fig. 66) and urinary obstruction (p. 39) are urogenital causes. Chronic leakage of amniotic fluid can produce the same results.

Features

Antenatally oligohydramnios, confirmed by ultrasound and also showing a compressed small-for-dates fetus. At birth, low-set ears, compression abnormalities with flexion contractures of limbs, and hypoplastic lungs. Possible renal failure with urogenital causes.

Course

Death is normally due to respiratory failure (pulmonary hypoplasia) soon after birth.

Ectopia vesicae (Fig. 68)

Incidence

Occurrences are very rare, although more common in males.

Features

Wide separation of public symphysis with ventral herniation of the bladder, exposure of bladder mucosa. It can be diagnosed antenatally with ultrasound and is often associated with rectal prolapse, together with renal and genital anomalies.

Management

Surgical reconstruction is difficult. Incontinence is common.

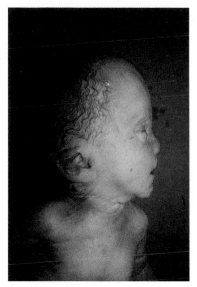

Fig. 65 Potter's facies.

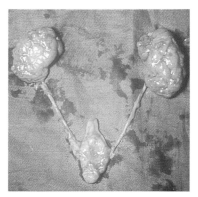

Fig. 66 Polycystic disease.

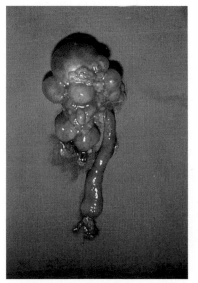

Fig. 67 Dysplastic kidney.

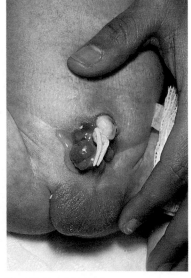

Fig. 68 Ectopia vesicae.

Congenital Abnormalities (5)

Renal tract anomalies (contd)

Urinary obstruction

Aetiology

Posterior uretural valves (males), congenital abnormalities of the urogenital system (such as a ureterocele) in females, pelvi-uteric obstruction.

Features

Antenatally, oligohydramnios may be seen, and severity depends on the site and extent of obstruction. On ultrasound, hydronephrosis may be seen (hydronephrosis may also be caused by reflux) (Figs. 69 and 70). When there is bladder outflow obstruction, there is also a grossly distended bladder (Figs. 71 and 72).

Management

This depends on the cause, the degree of renal impairment and the degree of oligohydramnios. If the obstruction is mild, the renal function is normal in at least one kidney, and the liquor volume is normal, then the pregnancy is allowed to continue; investigate and plan definitive treatment in the neonatal period. With severe oligohydramnios, the risk of Potter's syndrome (see p. 37) is high. If renal function is assessed as normal in one kidney (by fetal urinary electrolyte examination on urine obtained by ultrasound guided needling) then insertion of a vesico-amniotic shunt is possible in an attempt to preserve that kidney's function, restore liquor volume and prevent pulmonary hypoplasia. In many severe cases however, especially those presenting in the first half of pregnancy, renal function is irreparably damaged and the outlook is poor (Fig. 72).

OBSTETRICS

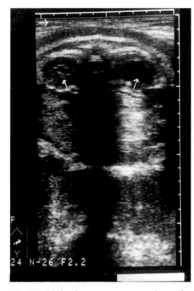

Fig. 69 U/S of transverse section of fetal abdomen (kidneys arrowed).

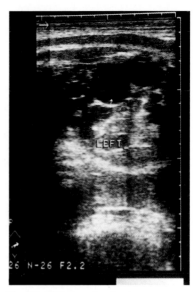

Fig. 70 U/S showing hydroureter (arrowed).

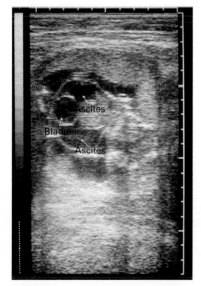

Fig. 71 U/S showing distended fetal bladder and urinary ascites.

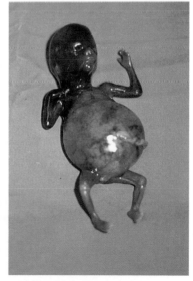

Fig. 72 Fetus with urethral valves and distended bladder.

Skeletal abnormalities

Osteogenesis imperfecta

Incidence
Uncommon. Varies in severity and inheritance. The severe congenital broad-boned type is autosomal recessive. Less severe forms may be autosomal dominant.

Features
Intrauterine diagnosis with ultrasound is possible. The long bones are deformed and shortened, and are poorly mineralized (as is the skull) with multiple fractures (Figs. 73 and 74). Rib involvement may produce respiratory compromise (Fig. 75).

Prognosis
Varies from perinatal death to survival beyond infancy, but usually with marked handicap (deformities and deafness from otosclerosis).

Short-limbed dwarfism

Incidence
Many causes and forms. Achondroplasia is the commonest (1 in 10 000 live births). Many are autosomal dominant (90% are fresh mutations). Severe forms (e.g. thanatophoric dwarfism—Fig. 76) are usually autosomal recessive.

Features
Short limbs, large head, prominent forehead. Severe forms have chest underdevelopment.

Prognosis
Milder forms: normal intelligence and life expectancy. *Severe forms:* neonatal death.

Limb reduction deformities
Some due to amniotic bands. Thalidomide taken in the first trimester causes shortened limbs (phocomelia) with rudimentary hands/feet or absent limbs (amelia). The cause for most today is unknown, although can be found in association with other abnormalities.

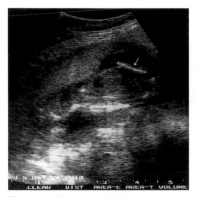

Fig. 73 U/S normal fetal femur (arrowed).

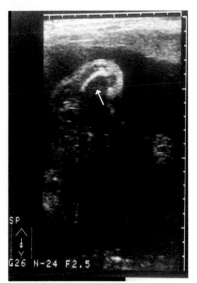

Fig. 74 U/S abnormal femur (shortening and angulation) (arrowed).

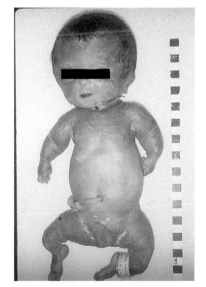

Fig. 75 Osteogenesis imperfecta.

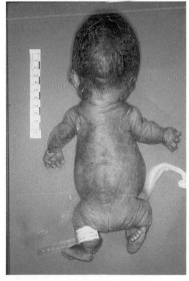

Fig. 76 Thanatophoric dwarfism.

Gastrointestinal anomalies

Diaphragmatic hernia

Incidence

Occurs in 1 in 1500 live births, and is caused by a failure of fusion or muscularization of the anterior and posterior leaves of the diaphragm.

Features

Antenatally: diagnosed on ultrasound (abdominal contents in the chest) (Fig. 77).
After birth: cardiorespiratory compromise with a scaphoid abdomen (Fig. 78). Clinical features and prognosis depend on the size of the hernia and degree of pulmonary hypoplasia (Fig. 79). Other abnormalities (chromosomal, gut) are found. Mortality is high (about 40%).

Tracheo-oesophageal fistula

Incidence

Occurs in 1 in 3000 live births. A developmental anomaly with the oesophagus ending in a blind upper pouch. Varying degrees of pathological communication with the trachea, bronchi or lower oesophagus.

Features

Hydramnios in 60% of cases. On ultrasound antenatally, a stomach bubble is consistently absent. If suspected, the baby should not be fed until a firm gastric tube has been passed to test for gastric acid (absent with atresia).

Prognosis

Depends on the degree and associated anomalies. Surgical correction is usually successful.

Intestinal obstruction

Hydramnios is found with obstruction beyond the oesophagus. Ultrasound may show either a 'double bubble' with duodenal atresia (the first bubble is the stomach and the second the distended proximal duodenum) or distended loops of bowel with peristalsis with more distal obstruction.

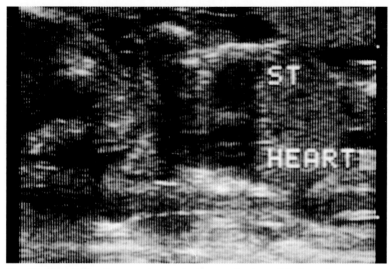

Fig. 77 U/S of diaphragmatic hernia (stomach alongside heart).

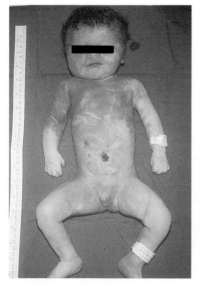

Fig. 78 Fetus with scaphoid abdomen.

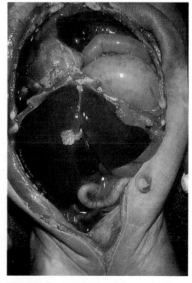

Fig. 79 Postmortem demonstration of diaphragmatic hernia.

9 | Rhesus Disease (1)

During pregnancy

Aetiology

Three allelic pairs of genes determine rhesus groups (C, D and E). The normal rhesus blood group is determined by the D locus. Rhesus (Rh) disease occurs when a Rh-negative mother has Rh antibodies and a Rh-positive baby. The antibodies cross the placenta and cause fetal haemolysis (anaemia, jaundice (Fig. 82)) and, in the extreme, cardiac failure as hydrops fetalis (Fig. 81) and death. Less severe disease can be produced by antibodies to the C or E loci, A, B or Kell antigens.

Sensitization

Occurs when Rh-positive cells enter the circulation of a Rh-negative woman (at delivery, abortion, placental bleeding, amniocentesis, CVS, external cephalic version or spontaneously).

Prevention

By administration of anti-D immunoglobulin to Rh-negative mothers at potential sensitization.

Detection

Unsensitized Rh-negative women are checked for antibodies during pregnancy.

Assessment

With antibodies, the severity of disease is given by amniotic fluid optical density difference at 450 nm (Fig. 80) and, in some centres, cordocentesis for fetal haemoglobin. The timing of these invasive procedures is determined initially by the maternal antibody level and then on the results.

Intervention

With mild or moderate disease (e.g. A), less frequent testing and delivery at term. With more severe disease (e.g. B), more frequent testing; if the prediction approaches the action line, either delivery for neonatal treatment (p. 47) if not too premature, or intrauterine transfusion of blood if extremely premature or if hydropic (Figs. 81, 84, 85 and 86).

OBSTETRICS

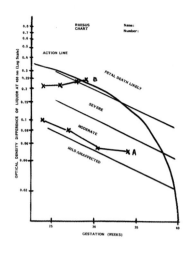

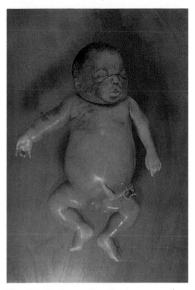

Fig. 80 Liley curve with examples of moderate (A) and severe (B) disease.

Fig. 81 Hydrops fetalis due to rhesus disease.

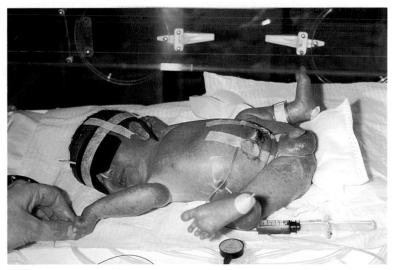

Fig. 82 Jaundiced newborn with rhesus disease; pigmented serum.

9 | Rhesus Disease (2)

In the newborn

Testing at birth

Cord blood is taken for haemoglobin, Coombs' test and bilirubin levels.

Risks to the newborn

1. *Haemolytic anaemia* (cardiac failure if severe).
2. *Jaundice* (Fig. 82) (kenicterus if unconjugated bilirubin levels are high).

Treatment

1. *Severe anaemia:* exchange transfusion and possible anti-failure treatment (e.g. with diuretics).
2. *Jaundice:* phototherapy in mild cases but exchange transfusion in severe cases.

10 | Hydrops Fetalis

See Figs. 83, 84, 85 and 86.

Causes

1. *Anaemia:* by haemolysis (Rh disease and incompatibility due to ABO, Kell and Duffy; red cell enzyme defects; homogygous α_1—thalassaemia) haemorrhage (twin-twin transfusion; fetomaternal haemorrhage) or marrow infiltration (Gaucher's disease).
2. *Cardiac failure:* arrhythmias, cardiac anomalies, cardiac tumours and arteriovenous shunts (fetal or placental).
3. *Hypoproteinaemia:* congenital nephrotic syndrome, hepatic enzyme defects.
4. *Obstructed venous return:* neuroblastoma, ovarian cysts, retroperitoneal fibrosis.
5. *Miscellaneous:* congenital infection (e.g. parvovirus), chromosomal anomaly (e.g. Turner's), chondrodystrophy.

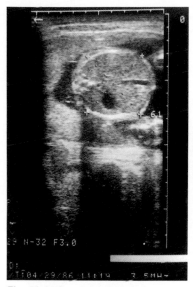

Fig. 83 U/S normal fetal abdomen (transverse).

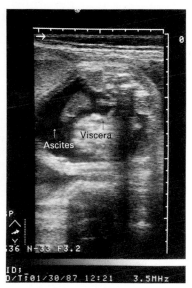

Fig. 84 U/S fetal ascites.

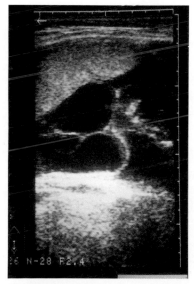

Fig. 85 U/S fetal head (compare with Fig. 59).

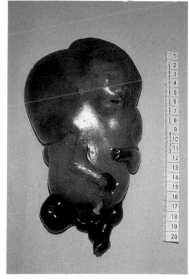

Fig. 86 Hydropic fetus.

11 | Maternal Disease (1)

Anaemia

Definition

Haemoglobin less than 10.5 g/dl.

Aetiology

'Physiological' (due to haemodilution) (Fig. 87), iron deficiency (hypochromic, microcytic, low-serum Ferritin) (Fig. 88) and folate deficiency (hyperchromic macrocytic, low red-cell folate) (Fig. 89). B_{12} deficiency, infection, haemoglobinopathies and other causes are uncommon.

Prophylaxis

In many women, the daily iron requirement cannot be met by the diet. For such mothers supplementation with iron (100 mg elemental iron/d) and folic acid (300 μg/d) is recommended. The use of iron and folate supplements for all mothers is controversial.

Investigations

Once the diagnosis has been made, other investigations undertaken include red cell indices (mean corpuscular volume, mean corpuscular haemoglobin concentration), reticulocyte count, film, serum ferritin, red-cell folate and serum B_{12} concentrations, and electrophoresis if a haemoglobinopathy is suspected.

Treatment

Depends on the cause. Mild 'physiological' anaemia requires no treatment. Iron and/or folate deficiency can be treated with oral iron and folic acid together. The use of parenteral iron (and oral folate) in hospital with its associated anaphylactic risks (rashes, arthralgia, angioneurotic oedema) should only be considered when all oral preparations have been unsuccessful. Blood transfusion in pregnancy should be a rare event (symptomatic severe anaemia).

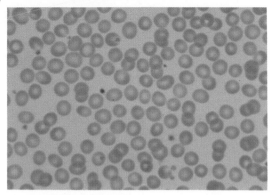

Fig. 87 Normal blood film.

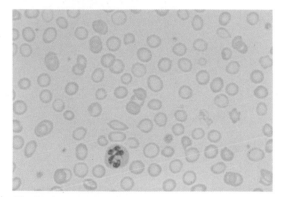

Fig. 88 Iron deficiency.

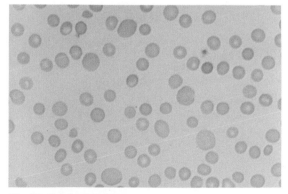

Fig. 89 Folate deficiency.

| # Maternal Disease (2)

Hypertension (HT)

Blood pressure measurement

Semirecumbent/sitting relaxed mother, upper arm level with heart (Fig. 90) and conventional sphygmomanometer (larger cuff with obese women—Fig. 91). The diastolic blood pressure (BP) is the point of muffling of the pulse (Korotkoff phase IV). Different equipment (Fig. 92) may produce significant differences in recordings.

Definition

A sustained absolute systolic BP of $\geqslant$140 mmHg or a sustained rise of $\geqslant$30 mmHg over booking values or a sustained absolute diastolic BP of $\geqslant$90 or a sustained rise of $\geqslant$15 mmHg over booking values.

Classification

1. Pregnancy induced HT (pre-eclampsia).
2. Pre-existing HT.
3. Pre-existing HT with added pre-eclampsia.

Definition

Pre-eclampsia
A condition peculiar to pregnancy of unknown aetiology, characterized by HT, renal impairment and fluid retention. Proteinuria and disseminated intravascular coagulation (DIC) may be found.

Types

1. *Mild* (10% of pregnancies): after 20 weeks, BP < 160/110, no proteinuria.
2. *Severe* (2% of pregnancies): after 20 weeks, BP $\geqslant$ 160/110, proteinuria ($\geqslant$ 0.5 g/l).

Associated factors

Primigravidity, previous severe pre-eclampsia, family history, pre-existing HT, migraine, low socio-economic status, multiple pregnancy and hydatidiform mole.

Causes

Pre-existing HT
Essential HT, renal HT, adrenal HT, connective tissue disorders, coarctation, drugs (oral contraceptives, steroids).

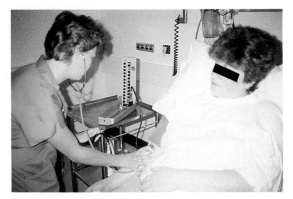

Fig. 90 Measuring blood pressure.

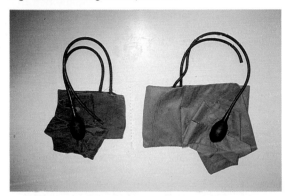

Fig. 91 Cuff size variation.

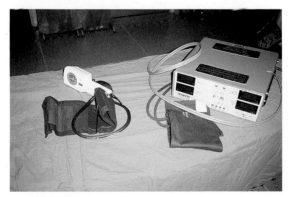

Fig. 92 Equipment variation.

11 | **Maternal Disease (3)**

Hypertension (HT) (contd)

Management

Mild HT (BP < 160/100, no proteinuria) managed as an outpatient; *severe HT* (with or without proteinuria) managed in hospital.

1. *Pre-eclampsia:* monitor condition, control BP if ≥160/100. Delivery is the only definitive cure. Relative indications are ≥37 weeks with growth retarded fetus and/or proteinuria. Absolute indications are uncontrollable HT, symptoms (occipital headaches, visual disturbance, epigastric pain due to liver capsule distension (Fig. 95), vomiting, brisk reflexes), eclampsia, renal or liver failure, DIC, and acute fetal compromise.
2. *Pre-existing HT:* monitor for pre-eclampsia supervening, control BP if ≥160/100.

Monitoring

BP, weight gain, symptoms; urine output are recorded (Fig. 93). Oedema (Fig. 94) is found with severe pre-eclampsia (but also in over 60% of normal pregnancies). Regular investigations include urine (protein content, bacteriology), serum uric acid (raised early in pre-eclampsia), urea and creatinine, platelet count, liver function tests. Assessment of fetal growth and health.

Drugs

To control BP: alpha-methyl-dopa, oxprenolol, atenolol, labetalol and nifedipine (oral) and hydrallazine and labetalol (intravenous). Drugs contra-indicated are angiotensin-converting enzyme inhibitors, diuretics (except with pulmonary oedema), sedatives and tranquillizers. Intravenous (i.v.) anti-convulsants used include diazepam and phenytoin.

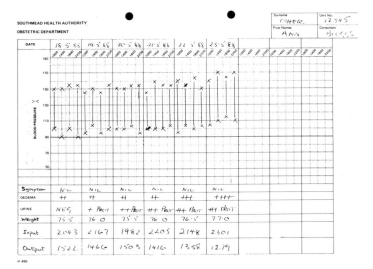

DATE	18·5·88	19·5·88	20·5·88	21·5·88	22·5·88	25·5·88			
Symptom	NIL	NIL	NIL	NIL	NIL	NIL			
OEDEMA	++	++	++	++	+++	++++			
URINE	NEG	+ Prot	++ Prot	++ Prot	++ Prot	++ Prot			
Weight	75·5	76·0	75·5	76·0	76·5	77·0			
Input	2043	2167	1982	2205	2148	2301			
Output	1522	1466	1503	1416	1338	1219			

M 485

Fig. 93 Pre-eclampsia chart.

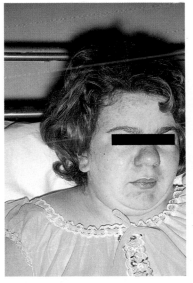

Fig. 94 Facial oedema.

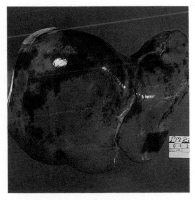

Fig. 95 Subcapsular hepatic haemorrhage.

| # Maternal Disease (4)

Diabetes mellitus

Risks

To mother: preterm delivery, HT, bleeding, traumatic delivery and/or Caesarean section, increased insulin requirements (Fig. 97).
To baby: congenital malformations (especially cardiac and musculoskeletal) (Fig. 98), macrosomia (Fig. 99), hydramnios, fetal death, respiratory distress, hypoglycaemia, jaundice and polycythaemia.

Prepregnancy

The aim is to improve periconceptual blood glucose control, reducing risk of congenital anomalies.

Gestational diabetes

More likely to develop in pregnancies complicated by glycosuria, a family history of diabetes, unexplained stillbirth, a previous baby weighing ≥90th centile, maternal obesity and hydramnios. More likely in pregnancies with raised random blood glucose (>6.9 mmol/l). However, an abnormal glucose tolerance test is required for definitive diagnosis.

Management

Close control of blood glucose (Fig. 96) (preprandial values 3−5 mmol/l, postprandial values ≤7 mmol/l). Some mothers may be managed on diet alone but most will require regular insulin; oral hypoglycaemics are contra-indicated. Regular checks of blood pressure and optic fundi. Fetal screening for normality at 16−18 weeks (alpha-feto-protein and scan) and later growth and health. Delivery (usually vaginal) at term in well-controlled, uncomplicated pregnancies. After delivery the insulin requirement falls.

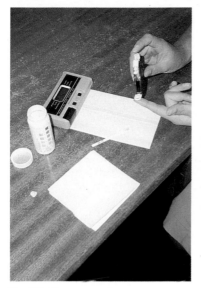

Fig. 96 Glucose testing.

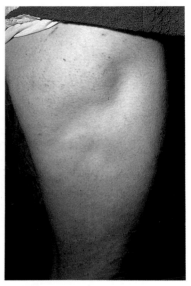

Fig. 97 Lipoatrophy of thigh associated with repeated insulin injections.

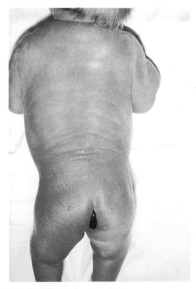

Fig. 98 Sacral agenesis.

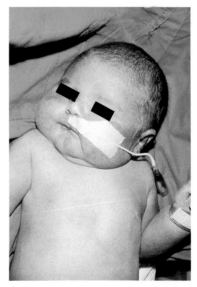

Fig. 99 Neonatal complications.

Infections (see also pp. 15–19)

Candidiasis
Commonest infection in pregnancy (fungus *Candida albicans*—Fig. 100). Usually presents as pruritus vulvae, white discharge and erythema. Wet films can be examined for mycelia and spores (Fig. 100). Treated with an anti-fungal agent (e.g. miconazole, clotrimazole).

Trichomoniasis
Trichomonas vaginalis produces pruritus and green frothy vaginal discharge. Microscopy of wet smears or culture confirms diagnosis. Oral metronidazole should be given to mother and male partner.

Gonorrhoea
Neisseria gonorrhoea (Fig. 101) attacks columnar and transitional epithelium (e.g. urethra, endocervix and anorectal canal). May be asymptomatic but usually presents with a purulent discharge from urethra or cervix. The baby can become infected during delivery and develop conjunctivitis (Fig. 102), arthritis, meningitis or generalized septicaemia. Treatment is with penicillin.

Urinary tract infection
Bacteriuria is significant when there are $>10^5$ organisms/ml of cultured urine (5% of pregnancies). Association with preterm delivery and anaemia. *E. coli* is the organism in 90% of cases. May present as (i) lower infection (asymptomatic or cystitis); outpatient treatment with oral antibiotics and liberal fluid intake is the treatment. (ii) upper infection (pyelonephritis); inpatient treatment with i.v. fluids and antibiotics is advisable.

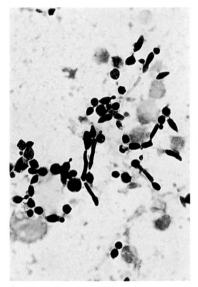

Fig. 100 *Candida albicans.*

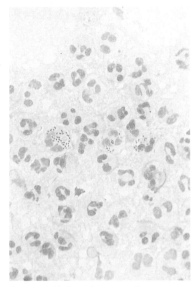

Fig. 101 Neisseria gonorrhoea.

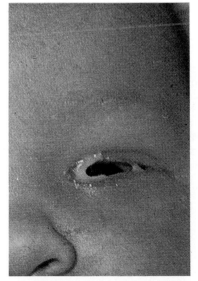

Fig. 102 Gonnococcal conjunctivitis.

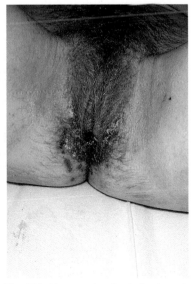

Fig. 103 Herpes simplex infection of genitalia.

Prescribed drugs

Most drugs both cross the placenta and are excrete
in breast milk. In the first trimester the theoretical
risk of congenital malformations is only proven
for a few drugs. Fetal growth and development
can be affected later (e.g. tetracycline-staining of
fetal teeth—Fig. 104; antithyroid agents and fetal
goitre—Fig. 105). Some drugs given close to term
or in labour can affect the newborn (e.g. narcotic
analgesia and neonatal depression). Drugs
should only be prescribed where there are clear
indications. Drug therapy in the first trimester
should be avoided if at all possible.

Smoking

Maternal smoking (20 cigarettes/day) reduces the
mean birthweight by 200–300 g. It is synergistic
with the effect of alcohol. It is prevented by
stopping smoking in the second half of
pregnancy.

Alcohol

Excessive chronic alcohol consumption ($\geqslant$80 g/d),
(10 g is a 0.5 pint, a 'short', a glass of wine or a
sherry) may cause the fetal alcohol syndrome
(Fig. 106): mental retardation, growth retardation,
characteristic facies with short palpebral fissures,
hypoplastic nasal philtrum and micrognathia.
Fetal growth retardation alone is a more
consistent finding with an alcohol consumption
of $\geqslant$40 g/d.

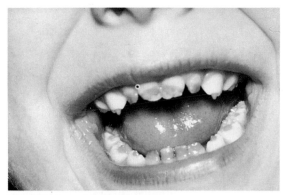

Fig. 104 Tetracycline teeth.

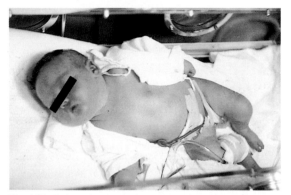

Fig. 105 Goitre due to maternal antithyroid treatment.

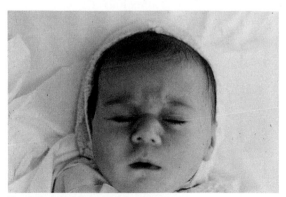

Fig. 106 Fetal alcohol syndrome.

| # Fetal Growth (1)

Intra-uterine growth retardation (IUGR)

General

10% of all live-born babies and 30% of those less than 2.5 kg suffer from intra-uterine growth retardation. They have greater perinatal mortality and morbidity and later handicap.

Definition

'When a baby fails to achieve his or her genetic growth potential.' In practice, however, the diagnosis is not always easy as there are ethnic and geographical variations. The best definition probably is where a baby's growth pattern or trajectory on ultrasound falls below that expected for the normal population.

Normal growth

Maximum velocity of linear growth occurs at 20 weeks, and of body weight at 34 weeks. At the end of pregnancy physical constraints probably slow fetal growth. Control is by genetic and hormonal factors and nutrient supply.

Causes

Intrinsic: malformations (5–10%) and viral infections (2%)
Extrinsic: uteroplacental vascular insufficiency (e.g. pre-eclampsia), cyanotic heart disease, maternal malnutrition if severe (e.g. in famines), smoking, alcohol and idiopathic causes (30%).

Risk factors

Short stature, previous small baby, low weight (<45 kg), poor weight gain, multiple pregnancy, smoking, alcohol, raised alpha-feto-protein, and other conditions (see *Causes*, above).

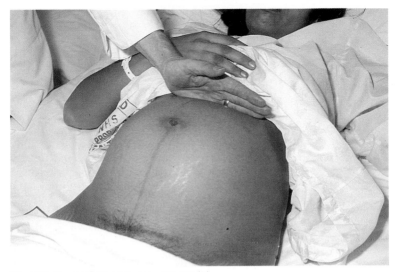

Fig. 107 Fundal height measurement (a).

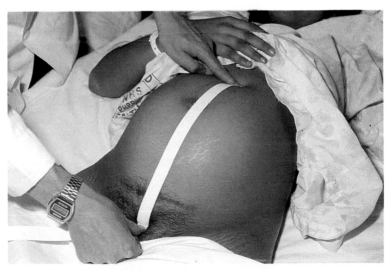

Fig. 108 Fundal height measurement (b).

Intra-uterine growth retardation
(contd)

Diagnosis

30–50% of IUGR fetuses remain undetected by clinical examination. Serial recording of symphysis-fundal height is claimed to be useful but this is not agreed by all (Figs. 107 and 108). Multiple pregnancy, polyhydramnios, transverse lie and maternal obesity reduce its accuracy. Assays of hormones (e.g. oestriol or placental lactogen) are no longer used widely. Ultrasound is the best method using the head and abdominal circumferences. Two patterns of IUGR are recognized:

1. *Symmetrical/early:* usually due to intrinsic problems (e.g. congenital abnormality, viral infection). On ultrasound, head *and* abdominal measurements fall away from expected growth trajectories (Fig. 109).
2. *Asymmetrical/late:* usually due to 'extrinsic' problems (e.g. pre-eclampsia, multiple pregnancy). On ultrasound, abdominal measurements fall away from expected growth trajectories *but* head circumference growth is initially normal (Fig. 110).

Management

The IUGR fetus should be scanned for congenital abnormality (p. 29). Cordocentesis (p. 23) for karyotyping or viral serology may be a necessary adjunct with severe cases. If normal then serial monitoring of fetal health is mandatory (pp. 65–67). The timing of elective delivery is determined by gestation and fetal health assessment.

Neonatal complications

Apart from major abnormalities, perinatal asphyxia, meconium aspiration, pulmonary haemorrhage, hypothermia, hypoglycaemia and polycythaemia.

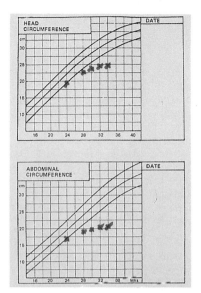
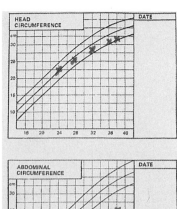

Fig. 109 Symmetrical/early fetal growth retardation.

Fig. 110 Asymmetrical/late fetal growth retardation.

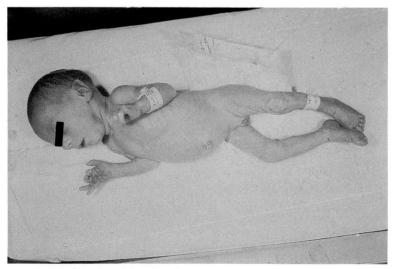

Fig. 111 Small-for-dates newborn.

13 | Fetal Health (Antepartum) (1)

Routine screening
Clinical assessment of fetal growth (Figs. 107 and 108) and noting maternal perception of fetal movements/activity. The fetal heart is also recorded routinely either by auscultation with a Pinard stethoscope (Fig. 112) or a fetal heart detector, using Doppler ultrasound (Fig. 113). The recording of the fetal heart in this way is a limited assessment of fetal welfare, being confined to answering the question of whether the fetal heart is present, and of normal rate at a given moment.

Additional methods
These methods are applicable to the fetus considered at risk either by using the above methods, because of a problem in a previous pregnancy (e.g. stillbirth), or because of ultrasonically diagnosed IUGR (pp. 61–63).
Biochemical assessment of fetal health (e.g. urinary or serum oestriol assays, plasma human placental lactogen) is no longer widely used because there is a delay between sampling and obtaining a result, and an overlap between normal and abnormal values; serial testing is usually advised and an accurate knowledge of gestational age is necessary.
Biophysical methods are more popular. The underlying principle is that the fetus exposed to a chronic hypoxic insult will have a depressed central nervous system (reduced heart rate variability, movements, tone and breathing movements and, if severe, depressed renal function (oligohydramnios)). The tests are the daily kick chart, non-stress fetal heart rate (FHR) recording (Fig. 114) and the biophysical profile (p. 67).

OBSTETRICS

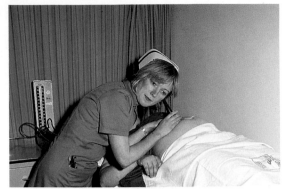

Fig. 112 Fetal heart auscultation with Pinard's stethescope.

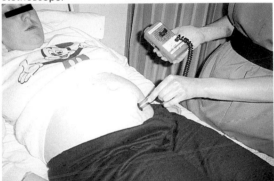

Fig. 113 Fetal heart auscultation with hand-held Doppler.

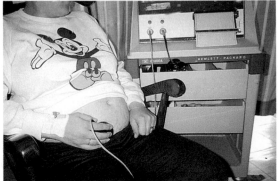

Fig. 114 Fetal heart rate recording technique.

Non-stress FHR monitoring
There is a close association between an abnormal FHR pattern and an asphyxiated fetus. The normal FHR trace at term is dependent on the state of the fetus. A fetus will be quiet for about 30% of the time (very little movements and a 'flat' trace—little oscillation of the baseline and no accelerations), and active for about 70% of the time (repeated movements and an 'accelerative' or 'reactive' trace—wide oscillations of the baseline and many accelerations of 15 beats per minute (bpm) or more). The presence of accelerations, a baseline rate of between 120–160 bpm and no decelerations (Fig. 115) is interpreted as reassuring of no evidence of asphyxia—in contrast to the fetus that is severely asphyxiated chronically (e.g. severe IUGR—Fig. 116) or acutely (e.g. placental haemorrhage—Fig. 117).

Biophysical profile scoring (BPS)
A more comprehensive assessment of the fetus at risk of asphyxia is provided by the BPS which records the presence of five biophysical variables: FHR pattern (non-stress test as above), fetal movements, fetal tone, fetal breathing and amniotic fluid volume. If four or five of these parameters are present in up to 30 minutes of recording then the risk of terminal fetal asphyxia is low.

Non-asphyxial causes of death
The biophysical methods of fetal assessment described above have only been shown to be valid for asphyxiated fetuses. Their value in other pathologies (e.g. metabolic or infective) is not established.

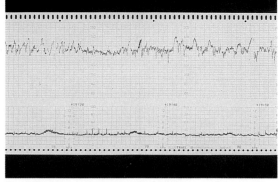

Fig. 115 Normal antepartum fetal heart rate recording at term.

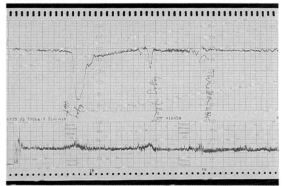

Fig. 116 Recording from asphyxiated growth retarded fetus.

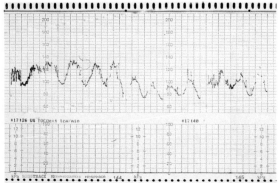

Fig. 117 Recording following abruptio placentae.

14 | Other Investigations

Kleihauer test
This detects fetal red blood cells (rbc) in maternal blood. Fetal rbc (containing haemoglobin-F) are less likely to haemolyse in alkaline pH than are maternal cells (containing haemoglobin-A). The test is used (i) after a potential sensitizing event in a rhesus-negative mother (p. 45) and (ii) to confirm a fetomaternal transfusion when there is a suspicion of concealed placental bleeding (p. 99).

X-rays
The use of X-rays in pregnancy has declined with the advent of ultrasound. It is used to measure the bony pelvis (pelvimetry) (Fig. 118) with, for example, a breech presentation at 37 weeks, suspected cephalopelvic disproportion, pelvic injury or disease and possible contraction (average anteroposterior diameters are: inlet 11.5 cm, midcavity 12.0 cm, outlet 12.5 cm). Plain X-rays are undertaken if there is a clinical indication. Contrast studies are avoided in pregnancy. If an intravenous pyelogram is performed after delivery, it is advisable for this to be deferred for 3 months so that the physiological changes of pregnancy have resolved (Fig. 119).

Doppler recording of blood flow
The use of Doppler ultrasound to record blood flow in maternal uterine and fetal circulations is a research tool at present. The absence of forward flow in diastoly in the umbilical arteries of a fetus with IUGR, however, is considered an ominous sign (Figs. 120 and 121).

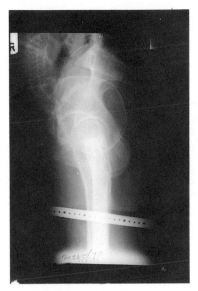

Fig. 118 X-ray pelvimetry.

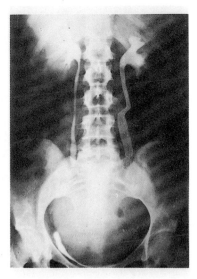

Fig. 119 Intravenous pyelogram—effects of pregnancy.

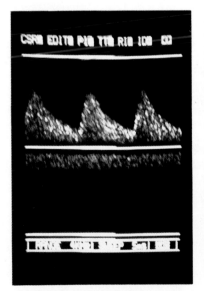

Fig. 120 Doppler recording from umbilical artery (normal).

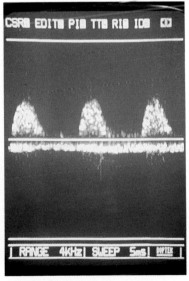

Fig. 121 Doppler recording from umbilical artery (absent end diastolic flow).

Onset

Definition

'The process of birth': characterized by (i) regular contractions; (ii) effacement and dilatation of the cervix and (iii) descent of the presenting part.

Onset

When regular uterine contractions and cervical changes begin. Diagnosis is not always easy (Braxton-Hicks contractions can be mistaken for labour; cervical effacement can predate dilatation by several days).

Diagnosis

1. Palpation of 'painful' regular contractions (Fig. 122), with a frequency of 1^+ in 5 minutes, a duration of 20^+ seconds.
2. Evidence of cervical effacement and/or dilatation (Fig. 123).
    The onset of labour is often associated with a 'show'—the passage vaginally of a blood-stained mucus plug from the cervix (Fig. 124). Membrane rupture (Fig. 125) is not necessary for the diagnosis of labour.

First stage

Definition

'From the onset of labour to full dilatation of the cervix.'
1. *Latent phase:* 'from the onset of labour to when the cervix is about 3 cm dilated and fully effaced'. Mean length in hours ($\pm$SD) is 9 ($\pm$6) in primigravidae and 5 ($\pm$4) in multigravidae.
2. *Active phase:* 'dilatation of the cervix from 3 cm'. The mean length in hours ($\pm$SD) is 5 ($\pm$3.5) in primigravidae and 2 ($\pm$1.5) in multigravidae.

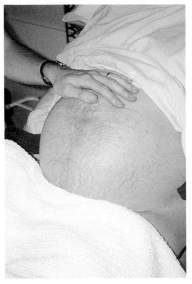

Fig. 122 Palpation of contraction.

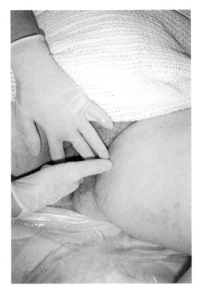

Fig. 123 Vaginal examination.

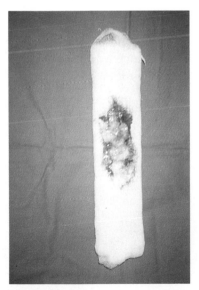

Fig. 124 'Show'.

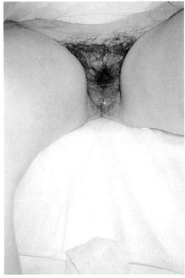

Fig. 125 Liquor draining from introitus under thighs and staining sheet.

15 | Labour (2)

Induction

Indications

The decision to end a pregnancy is because (i) the infant will be safer if delivered, or (ii) the risk to the maternal health of continuing with the pregnancy outweighs the risk to the baby of delivery. If the risk of labour is unacceptable, then delivery should be by Caesarean section. In other cases labour can be induced. Maternal indications may include hypertension, diabetes and cardiac disease. Fetal indications may include growth retardation, multiple pregnancy and premature rupture of the membranes at term.

Contra-ndications

1. *Absolute:* include a fetal lie that is not longitudinal and an insuperable obstruction to vaginal delivery.
2. *Extreme caution:* induction with grand multiparity, previous uterine scar.

Methods

1. Membrane rupture (amniotomy) with a amnihook (Fig. 126). This may have to be coupled with an i.v. infusion of an oxytocic agent, such as Syntocinon (Fig. 127).
2. Most inductions, however, are undertaken with prostaglandin-E_2 in many formulations (Fig. 128). The majority of inductions use vaginal tablets or pessaries, or gel. Vaginal delivery of a dead fetus or a fetus with a lethal malformation is more commonly undertaken using extra-amniotic preparations administered via an endocervical catheter.

Complications

Iatrogenic prematurity, hyperstimulation, infection, or failed induction. Large doses of Syntocinon can produce neonatal jaundice and water intoxication of mother and baby.

OBSTETRICS

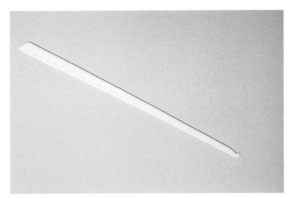

Fig. 126 Amnihook.

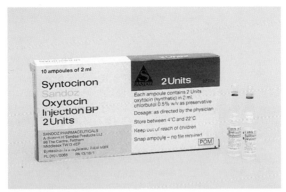

Fig. 127 Syntocinon.

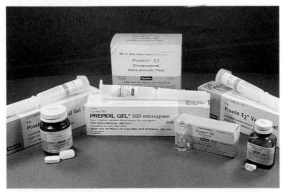

Fig. 128 Prostaglandins.

| # Labour (3)

Management

Preparation
Classes organized by midwives are available in most areas. Visits to hospital are usually arranged.

General principles
Overall conduct is the responsibility of a midwife alone or with reference to a general practitioner. An obstetrician need only be involved in those labours where problems are present (e.g. fetal distress, poor progress in labour, maternal disease).

Monitoring
Labour should be a normal event and management incorporates a programme of surveillance monitoring which confirms that it remains normal. There are three components of this monitoring, summarized on the partogram.
1. *Fetal condition* (Fig. 129): a record of the fetal heart rate recorded every quarter hour, colour of liquor drained vaginally and the degree of caput and/or moulding judged from vaginal examinations performed every 3–4 hours.
2. *Progress of labour* (Fig. 130): record of the descent of the head (assessed abdominally in fifths, and vaginally with respect to the ischial spines), the dilatation of the cervix on regular vaginal examinations, the strength and frequency of contractions and drugs given to augment/induce labour.
3. *Maternal condition* (Fig. 131): general well-being, pulse and blood pressure every half hour, temperature every 4 hours and fluid balance are recorded. All drugs given are noted. Urine passed is tested for glucose, protein and ketones.

OBSTETRICS

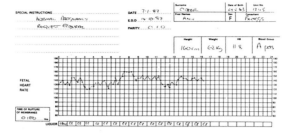

Fig. 129 Partogram—fetal section.

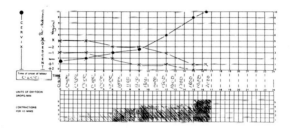

Fig. 130 Partogram—progress section.

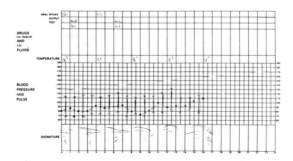

Fig. 131 Partogram—maternal section.

Fetal monitoring

Liquor
Normally the liquor is clear. Passage of meconium (Fig. 132) may be due to hypoxia and is an indication for continuous fetal heart rate (FHR) monitoring. Innocent causes are post-dates fetus and breech presentation. The baby is also at risk of meconium aspiration and requires expert care at birth. Mild blood staining may be just a 'show'. Heavier bleeding may be due to placental abruption, placenta praevia or vasa praevia (see pp. 97–99).

Moulding/caput
Severe degrees are significant, especially with poor progress (pp. 83–85) which may reflect cephalopelvic disproportion.

FHR monitoring
Routine: the fetal heart is normally recorded intermittently (every 15 minutes). The baseline should be between 120–160 bpm. Continuous FHR monitoring should be employed with pregnancies with an increased risk of intrapartum hypoxia, e.g. growth retardation, prematurity, breech presentation, multiple pregnancy, epidural analgesia, induced or augmented labour, diabetes, hypertension, bleeding, rhesus disease, auscultated FHR abnormalities, or meconium.
Continuous: the methods are (i) external Doppler recording (Fig. 133) or (ii) electrically triggered signals with a fetal skin electrode (Fig. 134). Inherent risks of skin electrodes (see p. 127) make an external transducer preferable (provided a good quality recording is obtained).

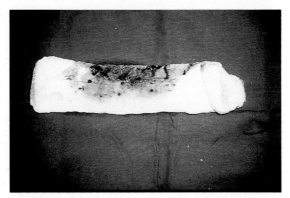

Fig. 132 Meconium.

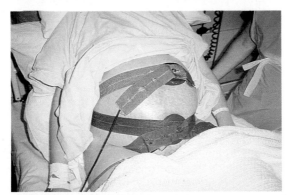

Fig. 133 External cardiotocography.

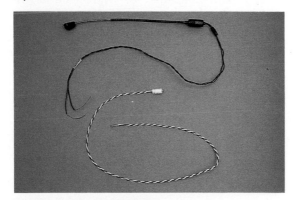

Fig. 134 Fetal scalp electrodes.

Fetal monitoring (contd)

FHR monitoring (contd)

Aim

Screening procedure for fetal hypoxia. Fetal hypoxia causes a rise of P_{CO_2}, a respiratory acidosis and an accumulation of lactate due to anaerobic glycolysis. The fetal blood pH falls. Interpretation of the significance of a FHR abnormality depends on the subsequent estimation of fetal pH by fetal blood sampling (FBS) (p. 81).

Fetal heart rates
Normal pattern (Fig. 135): baseline rate 120–160 bpm, variation of 5 or more bpm, no decelerations, acceleration with fetal movements or contractions.
Loss of baseline/short term variability (<5 bpm): can be seen with fetal hypoxia, (FBS indicated if prolonged) or maternal drug therapy (e.g. pethidine)
Baseline bradycardia (<120 bpm): low baselines (105–110 bpm) may be normal if postdates. Lower rates, especially if accompanied by other adverse features, are indications for FBS.
Fetal tachycardia (baseline rate >160 bpm, no accelerations): may be due to hypoxia thus FBS advisable. Also seen with maternal pyrexia.
Decelerations: (i) *Early* (Fig. 136) begins with contraction and returns to baseline by end of contraction; commonly due to change of pressure on fetal head (engagement, full- dilatation) (5% risk of low pH).
(ii) *Variable* (Fig. 137) variable in timing with respect to contraction, depth and duration; often due to cord compression (25% risk of low pH).
(iii) *Late* (Fig. 138) large deceleration of FHR after the contraction; commonly due to placental insufficiency (50% risk of low pH).

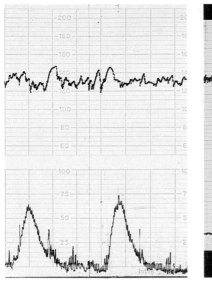

Fig. 135 Normal cardiotocograph.

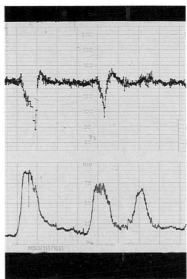

Fig. 136 Early decelerations.

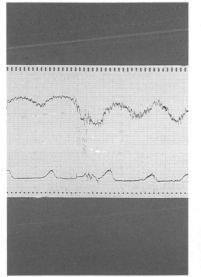

Fig. 137 Variable decelerations.

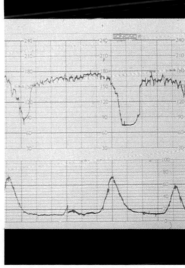

Fig. 138 Late decelerations.

Fetal monitoring (contd)

Fetal blood sampling (FBS)
With an abnormal FHR trace, turn mother on her left side, give oxygen by face mask, stop Syntocinon infusion (if present) and take FBS if abnormality persists.

Aim

To discover whether an abnormal FHR is due to fetal hypoxia and prevent severe asphyxia (white, apnoeic, hypotonic, bradycardic baby showing paucity of movement).

Equipment

pH meter, a cold light source, ethyl chloride spray, antiseptic lotions and cream, silicone jelly, small magnet with iron 'fleas' to stir the sample, and a pre-packed tray (Fig. 139) (amnioscopes, long instruments, 2 mm guarded blade, heparinized capillary tubes and swabs).

Procedure

The mother is placed in the left lateral position or in the lithotomy position with some lateral tilt, cleaned and gowned. An appropriately sized amnioscope is inserted through the cervix up against the fetal scalp (or buttocks if breech). The light source is attached. The fetal scalp is cleaned and a smear of silicone jelly applied. An assistant sprays the fetal scalp for 10 seconds to produce hyperaemia. The scalp is stabbed once with the guarded blade (Fig. 140). A continuous column of blood (10–30 μl), free of air bubbles, is collected in the capillary tube (Fig. 141). Pressure is applied to the fetal scalp to secure haemostasis.

Interpretation

pH >7.25 is normal; pH 7.20–7.25 is borderline, (repeat within 30 min); pH <7.20 is abnormal and delivery should be expedited.

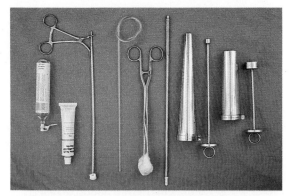

Fig. 139 Fetal scalp pH instruments.

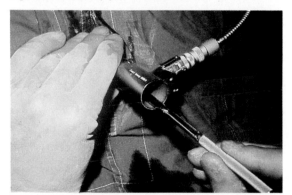

Fig. 140 Stabbing fetal scalp.

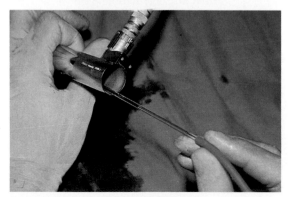

Fig. 141 Aspiration of fetal blood.

Progress

Normal progress in the first stage of labour
This has already been described (pp. 71–75) (Fig. 142). In primigravidae, delivery can be expected within 8 hours of the diagnosis of labour and should be achieved within 12 hours.

Delay in the first stage of labour

Causes

1. Inefficient uterine action (IUA)
2. Cephalopelvic disproportion (CPD) (either 'relative' due to occipitoposterior position (OPP) of fetal head, or 'absolute' due to large fetus and/or small maternal pelvis).

Patterns

1. Slow progress (Fig. 143) which is more commonly, although not always, found with IUA.
2. Secondary arrest (Fig. 144) which is more commonly, although not always, found with CPD.

Management

1. What is the cause of the delay? Is there evidence of CPD (e.g. short mother, large baby, late engagement of fetal head, OPP)? Is there clinical evidence of IUA?

If it is possible that the cause is IUA and potentially correctable then:

2. Correct any ketosis/dehydration with oral or i.v. fluids.
3. Rupture the membranes.
4. If these measures are not successful then augmentation of labour should be considered (see p. 85).
5. Evaluation of effect of management.

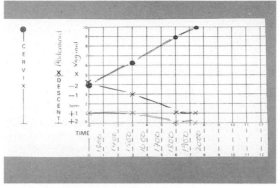

Fig. 142 Partogram—normal progress.

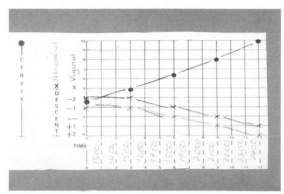

Fig. 143 Slow progress.

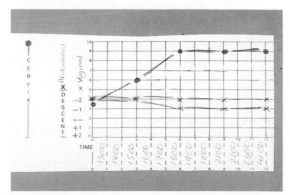

Fig. 144 Secondary arrest.

Progress (contd)

Augmentation of labour (see also p. 83).
The normal method is with a Syntocinon infusion (start at 2 mU/min and double every 20 min to a maximum of 32 mU/min until progress is achieved). Augmentation in a multiparous mother should be only undertaken after careful consideration by an experienced obstetrician (due to greater risk of uterine rupture). The use of an intrauterine pressure catheter (IUPC) (see below) may permit a more objective augmentation policy in certain cases.

Evaluation of management of delay
Once delay has been recognized and a management plan (p. 83) implemented, the effect of the management on the progress of labour is critically reviewed after 2–3 hours. If the rate of progress has not been improved then Caesarean section may have to be performed.

Contractions
Manual palpation is normally used to evaluate uterine activity; it is not a direct method. An IUPC measures pressure directly (Figs. 145, 146 and 147). Indications for use of this invasive procedure include management of augmented labour with possible CPD or a uterine scar. Between contractions the intrauterine pressure is usually <10 mmHg and at the peak of effective contractions, about 50 mmHg.

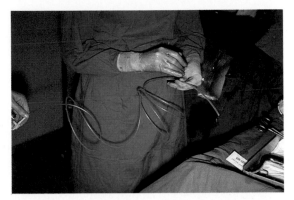

Fig. 145 Water-filled IUPC.

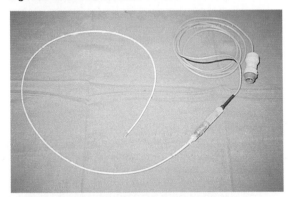

Fig. 146 Gaeltec catheter IUPC.

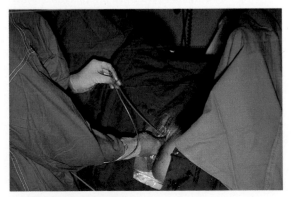

Fig. 147 Insertion IUPC.

Maternal condition

General

As far as possible, labour should be both safe for mother and baby and also an emotionally rewarding experience. Mobility should be encouraged during the latent phase of labour (Fig. 148).

Analgesia

The mother should decide whether she wants pain relief in labour, although the availability may vary. Ambulation (Fig. 148) and the presence of a supportive partner (Fig. 149) are helpful. Psychological/relaxation methods may help. Antenatal education is an integral part of the process.

Inhalational agents: nitrous oxide (50%) and oxygen (50%) as 'Entonox' (Fig. 149) are used by the mother often towards the end of the first stage and during the early part of the second stage. Longer administration is not practical. They are effective and safe for mother and baby.

Transcutaneous nerve stimulator (Fig. 150): this is usually only effective in early labour and with relatively mild contractions.

Opiates: intramuscular pethidine (50–150 mg) with or without a phenothiazine is the most widely used method of pain relief in Britain. The advantages of opiates are ease of administration, rapid effect, low incidence of serious side-effects and antagonists are available. The disadvantages include inadequate analgesia in 40%, vomiting is common and neonatal respiratory depression.

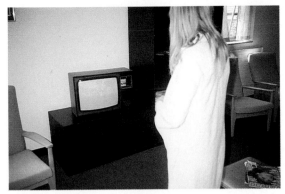

Fig. 148 Ambulation.

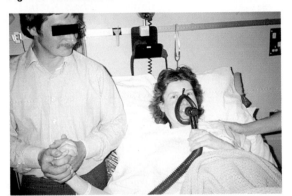

Fig. 149 Entonox and partner.

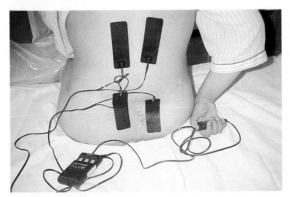

Fig. 150 Transcutaneous nerve stimulator.

Maternal condition (contd)

Epidural analgesia
This is the most effective analgesic method but experience in its use is essential.

Indications

On request, IUA, OPP, prolonged labour, breech presentation, multiple pregnancy, preterm labour, forceps delivery, hypertension, maternal distress/exhaustion.

Contra-indications

Lack of experienced personnel, infection at insertion site, spinal abnormalities, coagulation abnormalities, hypovolaemia. Careful monitoring is necessary with a previous Caesarean section scar.

Complications

Dural puncture (headache), total spinal block (loss of sensory and motor function, unconsciousness, hypotension, apnoea), hypotension (due to caval compression, reduced venous return and cardiac output, and pooled blood in splanchnic bed), motor paralysis, urinary retention, toxic reactions.

Management

The materials used are prepacked (Fig. 151). Insertion is in the left lateral or upright positions (Figs. 152 and 153). The cannula is strapped over one shoulder for ease of access (Fig. 154), with a bacterial filter. An i.v. infusion of Hartmann's solution is first established (to correct any hypotension). Bupivicaine (repeated injections for continuous analgesia) or lignocaine (single injection) are used. The dose (8–12 ml) is tailored to the patient. BP, respirations and FHR (continuous) are carefully monitored.

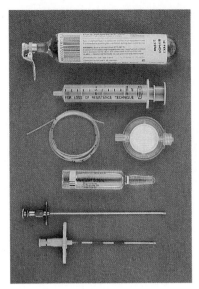

Fig. 151 Epidural—kit.

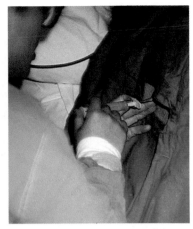

Fig. 152 Epidural—insertion (a).

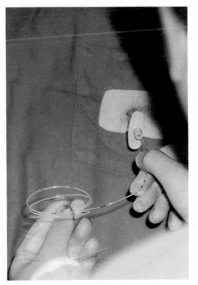

Fig. 153 Epidural—insertion (b).

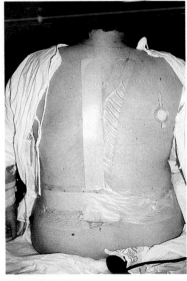

Fig. 154 Epidural—in use.

Second stage

Definition

From full dilatation of the cervix to delivery of the baby. Average duration is 40 minutes in primigravidae and 20 minutes in multiparae.

Phases

1. *Propulsive:* from full dilatation to the presenting part reaching the pelvic floor.
2. *Expulsive:* from then until the birth of the baby. The mother wishes to push or 'bear down' and the perineum is distended.

Management

A mother should not normally be encouraged to push until the head is visible and/or the perineum is distended (Fig. 155). The decision to perform an episiotomy requires considerable experience and judgement (see also pp. 101–103). The aim of an episiotomy is to deliver the fetal head avoiding severe perineal tear. However, not all mothers will experience a severe perineal tear and certainly most multiparae will be able to have a delivery with an 'intact perineum'. Primigravidae also may be able to avoid an episiotomy ('episiotomy for all primigravidae' should be discouraged). If episiotomy is necessary then the perineum initially is infiltrated with 10 ml 1% lignocaine as it is distended (Fig. 156). The episiotomy (extending from the fourchette, posterolaterally) is performed during a contraction when the perineum is maximally distended (Fig. 157). The delivery of the fetal head ('crowning') is controlled with the left hand on the vertex and the right hand applying a pad to the perineum (Fig. 158).

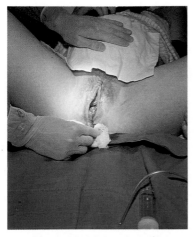

Fig. 155 Head visible at introitus.

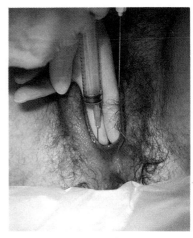

Fig. 156 Infiltration of perineum with local anaesthetic.

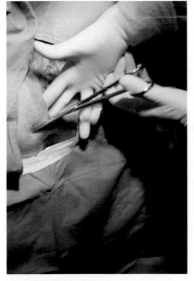

Fig. 157 Episiotomy.

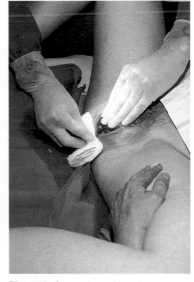

Fig. 158 Crowning of head.

Second stage (contd)

The left hand (Fig. 159) prevents too rapid a delivery and decompression of the fetal head (especially important in the preterm infant). The right hand (Fig. 159) prevents uncontrolled tearing of the perineum. Once the head is delivered the face is wiped with a clean swab. A hand is inserted to check for the presence of the cord around the baby's neck (Fig. 160). If found, it is either clamped and cut or pulled over the head. Whilst the head is on the perineum it usually rotates to realign with the axis of the shoulders. The mother pushes again and, with the hands placed over the baby's parietal eminences, gentle traction is applied posteriorly to encourage the delivery of the anterior shoulder (Fig. 161). Anterior traction is then applied and the posterior shoulder and the body are delivered. An intramuscular injection of an oxytocic agent is given with the delivery of the anterior shoulder (p. 95). Once the baby is delivered the cord is double-clamped and cut. The baby is dried and wrapped (Fig. 162), checked to ensure that he or she is breathing normally and handed to the mother. The baby will later be cleaned, dressed and placed in a cot.

Apgar score is traditionally used to record the condition of the baby at birth (at 1, 5 and 10 min) using five parameters: heart rate, respiratory effort, muscle tone, response to stimulation and colour, each scored 0, 1 or 2).

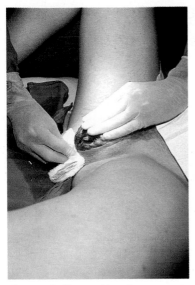

Fig. 159 Delivery of head.

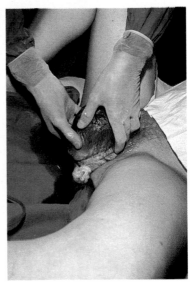

Fig. 160 Check for cord.

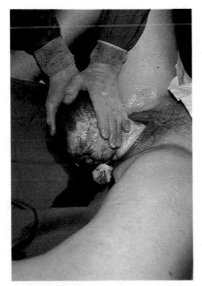

Fig. 161 Delivery of shoulders.

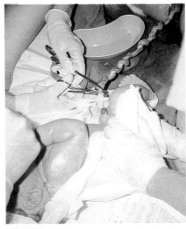

Fig. 162 Drying and wrapping baby and clamping cord.

Third stage

Definition

This begins with delivery of the baby and ends when the placenta is delivered.

Management

1. *Active* (most common form in UK): administration of an oxytocic agent (intramuscular (i.m.) Syntometrine containing 5 units Syntocinon and 0.5 mg ergometrine or i.m. Syntocinon 10 units) with the delivery of the anterior shoulder (p. 93); clamping and cutting the cord (Fig. 162) and delivery of the placenta once there are signs of separation (contraction of the uterus, a gush of blood (Fig. 163) and descent/'lengthening' of the cord). The placenta and membranes are delivered by controlled cord traction (Figs. 164 and 165).
2. *Passive:* no oxytocic agent, no cord clamping and waiting for the spontaneous delivery of the placenta. Higher incidence of primary postpartum haemorrhage.

Primary postpartum haemorrhage
(5% incidence)
'The loss of 500 ml of blood or more within 24 hours of delivery'. Causes include retained placenta (whole or part), hypotonic uterus, trauma (uterine rupture, cervical or vaginal lacerations), multiple pregnancy, large baby and clotting disorder. The two principles of management are (i) resuscitation measures, and (ii) to identify and treat the cause. An examination under anaesthetic may be necessary if the cause is uncertain. Internal iliac artery ligation or hysterectomy may be necessary on rare occasions.

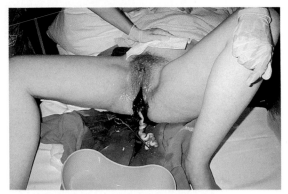

Fig. 163 Blood flow and contraction.

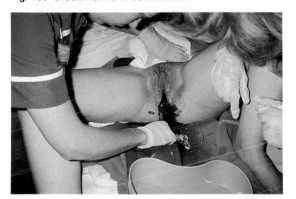

Fig. 164 Controlled cord traction.

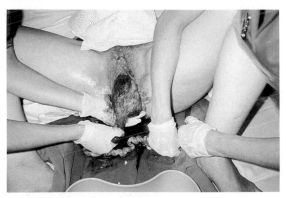

Fig. 165 Delivery of placenta.

16 | Placenta (1)

Early development
Implantation of the blastocyst occurs approximately 6 or 7 days following fertilization. The solid inner cell mass forms the fetus, whilst the cyst wall becomes the trophoblast. The trophoblast differentiates into an inner layer (cytotrophoblast) and an outer layer (syncytiotrophoblast). The endometrium becomes decidua (Fig. 166). By the 14th day the trophoblast has developed into chorionic villi with a central core of mesenchyme. The villi eventually disappear from the surface of the blastocyst except in the area adjacent to the uterus; this will form the placenta. During the second trimester, the syncytiotrophoblast degenerates and the normal haemochorial circulation is formed.

Functions of the placenta
These are respiratory (gas exchange), nutritional (food and waste products), protein production (oestrogen, progesterone, hCG, human placental lactogen and other placental proteins).

Pathology
1. *Morbid adherence (placenta accreta)* (Fig. 167): the placenta implants into the myometrum. It is a cause of retained placenta and post partum haemorrhage (PPH). Uncontrollable haemorrhaging may necessitate hysterectomy.
2. *Infection (chorioamnionitis)* (Fig. 168): associated with prolonged rupture of the membranes and fetal death.
3. *Succenturiate lobe* (Fig. 169): the placenta is in two parts linked by communicating vessels.
4. *Velamentous insertion:* cord divides and crosses the membranes to the placenta.

OBSTETRICS

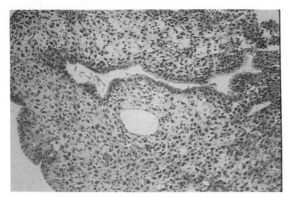

Fig. 166 Normal decidua.

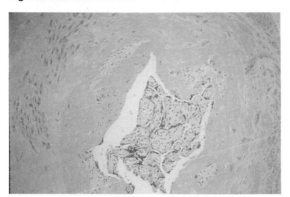

Fig. 167 Placenta accreta.

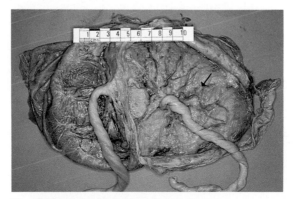

Fig. 168 Amnionitis in one of twin placentas (arrowed).

Pathology (contd)
5. *Multiple pregnancy* (Fig. 170): there can be a pathological communication.
6. *Antepartum haemorrhage* (see below).

Antepartum haemorrhage

Definition

'Bleeding from the genital tract from 28 weeks and before delivery of the baby'.

Causes

1. *Placenta praevia:* bleeding from placenta encroaching into the lower uterine segment. Usually painless.
2. *Placental abruption:* bleeding from a normally situated placenta. Usually painful. Amount of blood passed vaginally can vary.
3. *Vasa praevia:* bleeding from a ruptured vessel in the membranes. Often occurs following amniotomy.
4. *'Show':* at the onset of labour.
5. *Bleeding from other sites.*

Management

1. Assess blood loss and resuscitate.
2. The fetal condition should be assessed.
3. Establish cause. A vaginal examination should be avoided until the placental site is known.
4. If the bleeding ceases and the fetus is healthy, a placenta praevia is managed as inpatient (close to emergency Caesarean section and blood transfusion available promptly), other causes are managed as outpatients.
5. If the bleeding continues the delivery should be expedited, the route chosen (vaginal or abdominal) depending on the amount of bleeding, gestation and fetal health.

Value of placental examination after delivery This is variable: it is unhelpful in, e.g. IUGR and pre-eclampsia but useful in, e.g. lost IUCD (Fig. 171), infection, and multiple pregnancy.

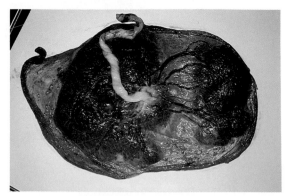

Fig. 169 Succenturiate lobe.

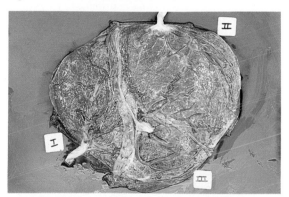

Fig. 170 Triplet placentae.

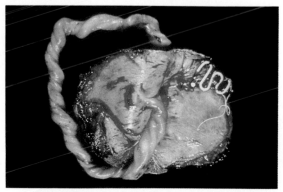

Fig. 171 Intra-uterine contraceptive device in placenta.

Indications for episiotomy

The decision to perform an episiotomy should never be 'routine', but rather a matter for experienced clincial judgement. Possible indications include:
1. Avoidance of inevitable severe perineal tear.
2. Fetal distress late in second stage.
3. Most forceps deliveries (to avoid tears).
4. Breech delivery.

The episiotomy (posterolateral) should be performed with sharp scissors at the correct time (too early results in unnecessary blood loss, while too late may end with a perineal tear anyway), with adequate analgesia (local or regional) and repaired properly as quickly as possible after delivery.

Technique

The patient is placed in the lithotomy position and the vulva and perineum cleaned and gowned. There should be adequate analgesia using local anaesthetic (Fig. 172) or regional analgesia.
Vaginal skin: the apex of the vaginal incision must be clearly identified (Fig. 173). The vaginal skin is repaired with a continuous suture of either chromic catgut or polyglycolic acid, starting just above the apex of the incision (Fig. 174). Care must be taken to ensure an even apposition of the vaginal skin edges. The suture is tied at the level of the Carunculae myritiformes (remnants of the hymen).
Perineal tissues: on completion of the vaginal suturing the defect in the perineum should be approximately elliptical (Fig. 175). The deep tissues of the perineum are repaired with interrupted sutures of either chromic catgut or polyglycolic acid (Fig. 176).

OBSTETRICS

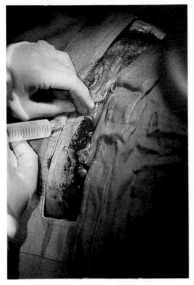

Fig. 172 Infiltration with local anaesthetic.

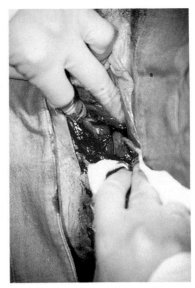

Fig. 173 Inspection of apex of vaginal incision.

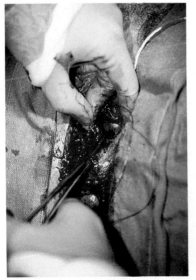

Fig. 174 Vaginal suture.

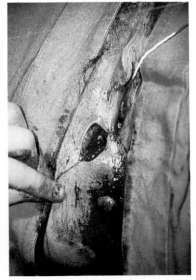

Fig. 175 Unsutured perineal body.

Perineal tissues (contd). The perineal body sutures (Fig. 176) are inserted with care to avoid penetration of the rectum and at right angles to the axis of the defect.

Perineal skin: the perineal skin is repaired with either chromic catgut or polyglycolic acid sutures. Interrupted sutures (Fig. 177) or a subcuticular technique may be used. After the repair has been completed a vaginal examination is performed (Fig. 178) to check that no swabs have been left in the vagina and that there is no remaining defect or haematoma. Finally, a rectal examination is performed to confirm that no sutures have penetrated the rectal mucosa (Fig. 179).

After-care

Adequate analgesia should be offered to the mother, both systemic (oral analgesics) and topical (ice-packs, haemalis water).

First degree (skin only) and second degree (skin and perineal body) perineal tears are managed and repaired in the same way.

Third degree tear is a tear which extends to include the rectum and/or the anal sphincter. It is repaired in theatre under general or regional anaesthesia by an experienced obstetrician. The rectum and anus are first repaired with interrupted chromic catgut sutures (knots in rectal lumen) and then the edges of the sphincter are apposed and sutured. The residual second degree tear is repaired separately afterwards. The mother is given a high fibre diet and aperient afterwards.

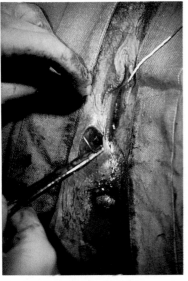

Fig. 176 Perineal body suture.

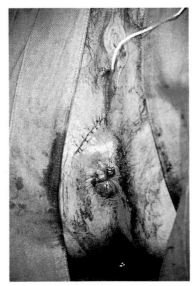

Fig. 177 Sutured skin.

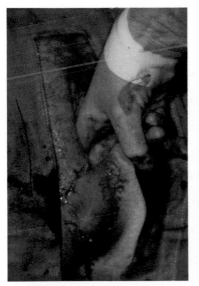

Fig. 178 Vaginal examination.

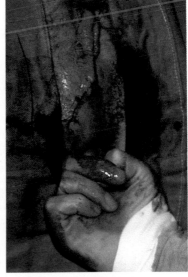

Fig. 179 Rectal examination.

18 | Forceps (1)

Prerequisites

1. A valid indication must exist (see below).
2. Suitable presentation.
3. No cephalopelvic disproprotion and no excessive moulding.
4. Engaged head and ideally no fetal head palpable per abdomen.
5. Known position of the fetal head.
6. Full dilatation of the cervix.
7. Adequate analgesia.
8. Empty bladder.
9. Adequate uterine contractions.

These requirements apply to use of the ventouse (p. 109), except that it may be used before full cervical dilatation (9 cm or more).

Indications

1. Maternal conditions where prolonged expulsive efforts may be contra-indicated, e.g. cardiac disease, hypertension, dural tap.
2. Fetal distress in the second stage.
3. Cord prolapse in the second stage.
4. Poor progress in the second stage due to maternal exhaustion or occipitoposterior position.

Types

1. *Non-rotational:* suitable for occipito-anterior positions of the fetal head (A in Fig. 180). They have a cephalic curve and a pelvic curve (e.g. Rhodes, Wrigleys, Simpsons).
2. *Rotational:* suitable for transverse or occipito-posterior positions (B in Fig. 180). They only have a cephalic curve (e.g. Kiellands).

Procedure

Non-rotational: after abdominal palpation, the mother is placed in the lithotomy position, cleaned, gowned and catheterized (Fig. 181). A vaginal examination is performed to confirm full dilatation; check the position and station, and assess pelvic capacity (Fig. 182).

OBSTETRICS

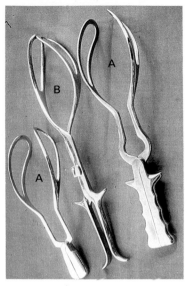

Fig. 180 Variation in forceps.

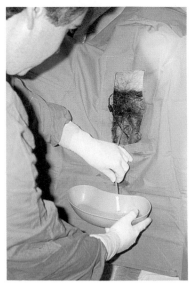

Fig. 181 Preparation.

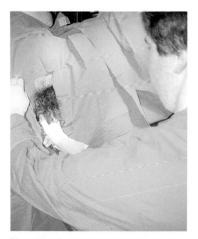

Fig. 182 Vaginal examination.

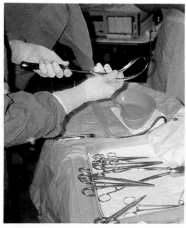

Fig. 183 Lubricating forceps.

Procedure
(contd)

Analgesia must be adequate: regional analgesia (e.g. epidural) or local anaesthetic with 1% lignocaine (pudendal and perineal blocks). The forceps blades are lubricated (Fig. 183) and guided alongside the fetal head (left blade first) (Fig. 184). Traction is applied with a contraction and maternal effort (Fig. 185). An episiotomy is normally performed and the head delivered gently with protection of the perineum as for a normal delivery (Fig. 186). The forceps blades are removed (Fig. 187). The remainder of the delivery is as for a normal delivery (p. 93).

Occipitoposterior delivery ('Face to pubes'): in certain cases it may be preferable to deliver in the occipitoposterior position without rotation (e.g. deeply engaged head, or pelvis with narrow transverse diameter inhibiting rotation). This method of delivery requires great judgement, experience and skill.

Forceps for delivery of the head with a breech presentation: this method allows control of the delivery preventing intracranial trauma.

Forceps for delivery of low birth weight (LBW) infants: there is no evidence that elective forceps delivery of LBW infants confers any benefit on the baby.

Trial of forceps: this term refers to those cases where it is considered likely, although not totally certain, that vaginal delivery by forceps will be successful. A trial of forceps must be carried out by an experienced obstetrician in a theatre prepared for immediate Caesarean section.

OBSTETRICS

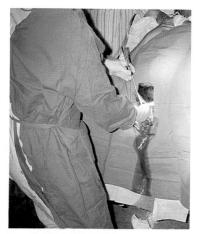

Fig. 184 Applying blade.

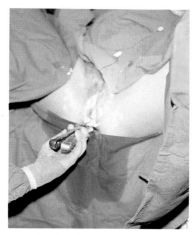

Fig. 185 Traction.

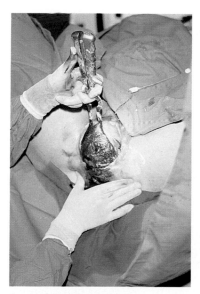

Fig. 186 Head crowning.

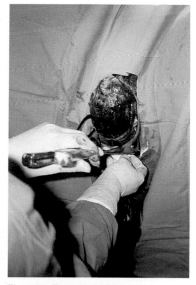

Fig. 187 Removal of forceps.

19 | Ventouse

Indications

Same as for forceps.

Instruments
Stainless steel or plastic cup, diameter varies (30 mm, 40 mm or 50 mm) with size of baby's head, and a chain and suction tube (Fig. 188).

Technique

A suitably sized cup is applied as near to the occiput as possible (to maintain flexion during traction) (Fig. 189) and a vacuum is created by means of a hand or electric pump (Fig. 190). The pressure is initially increased to 0.2 kg/cm^2 and having checked there is no vagina or cervix included under the rim, the pressure is gradually increased to 0.8 kg/cm^2. This draws the scalp into the cup in the shape of a chignon or bun. Traction is then applied to the chain coinciding with uterine contractions and maternal pushing and when the head passes through the introitus, the suction is released (Fig. 191).

Complications

Fetal scalp abrasions (Fig. 215, p. 123) and cephalhaematomas (Fig. 214, p. 123) are common. Retinal haemorrhages, intracranial haemorrhage and scalp necrosis rarely occur. Fetal haemorrhage may result if the cup is applied following fetal blood sampling.

Advantages
The ventouse can be applied near to full dilatation, and used for either low cavity or midcavity extraction where rotation of the fetal head is required. For the latter indication, it is easier to learn than rotational forceps, requires less analgesia and carries less risk of maternal trauma.

Disadvantages
Delivery time is prolonged (and so method is inappropriate if there is fetal distress); it is relatively inefficient in cases of malrotation. It cannot be used in cases of face presentation or in a breech delivery for delivering the head.

OBSTETRICS

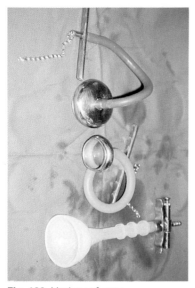

Fig. 188 Variety of cups.

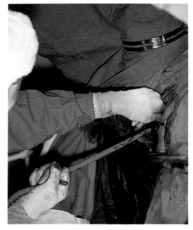

Fig. 189 Application of cups.

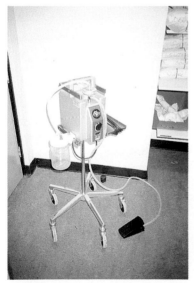

Fig. 190 Suction machine.

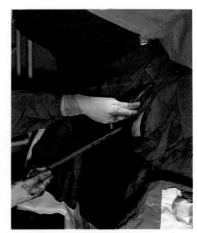

Fig. 191 Traction.

Incidence

Varies with policies of different centres. Currently 10–15% in UK and 20–25% in North America. May be elective (planned in advance) or an emergency. Maternal and perinatal mortality and morbidity are higher when the operation is an emergency.

Indications

Routine CS
1. Previous CS for recurrent cause (e.g. small pelvis).
2. Two or more previous CS.
3. Breech presentation with small pelvis, and/or big baby, and/or footling presentation (increased risk of cord prolapse).
4. Placenta praevia.

Indications

Emergency CS
1. Fetal distress (abnormal cardiotocography, acidosis, cord prolapse or abruption) before or during the first stage of labour.
2. Obstructed labour (e.g. pelvic cyst/fibroid).
3. Prolonged labour due to dysfunctional uterine activity or disproportion.
4. Bleeding from placenta praevia.
5. Preterm delivery with estimated fetal weight <1000 g but where there is prospect of viability (controversial).
6. Preterm breech delivery where the estimated weight is 1000–1500 g.
7. Delivery for maternal risk (e.g. uncontrollable HT, eclampsia) where prompt vaginal delivery is not feasible (usually preterm).

Technique up to incision

Following induction of general or regional anaesthesia the patient is catheterized, and the abdomen is cleaned with antiseptic (Fig. 192) and draped with sterile towels. The abdomen is opened with either a lower transverse incision (Fig. 193) or a midline subumbilical incision.

OBSTETRICS

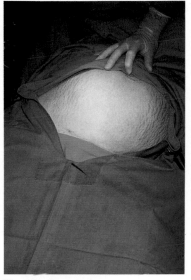

Fig. 192 Preparation.

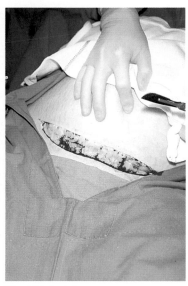

Fig. 193 Incision.

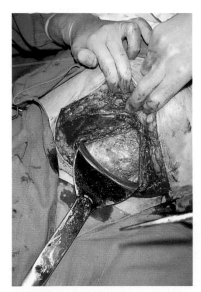

Fig. 194 Exposure of lower uterine segment.

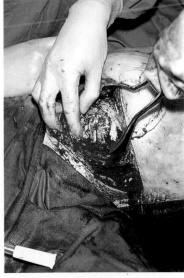

Fig. 195 Delivery of head (forceps)

Types of operation

1. *Lower segment:* this is the commonest approach, used in 99% of cases. Uterovesical peritoneum is reflected (Fig. 194) and the lower segment opened with a transverse incision. The risk of rupture in subsequent labour is low (about 0.1%).
2. *Upper segment:* this approach was used for several centuries, hence its description as 'classical'. Vertical incision is made in the upper segment of the uterus. Greater blood loss, higher risk of rupture in a subsequent labour (4–9%), and greater risk of bowel adhesions and post-operative ileus.

Note: the type of previous CS cannot be determined from the skin incision.

Indications for classical CS

1. Transverse lie which cannot readily be converted to longitudinal (e.g. prolapsed arm).
2. Certain uterine abnormalities, e.g. fibroids in the lower segment.
3. Some cases of placenta praevia.
4. For delivery of some low birth weight babies, particularly with oligohydramnios (poorly formed lower segment where delivery may be difficult and traumatic).
5. Dense adhesions obscuring the lower segment.

Technique after incision

The head is delivered either manually or with forceps (Figs. 195 and 196). Syntocinon is administered i.v. to the mother and the placenta delivered by cord traction (Fig. 197). the uterus is repaired in two layers of continuous absorbable sutures (Fig. 198). The abdomen is closed in layers (Fig. 199). Post-operative attention is paid to analgesia, physiotherapy, mobilization and assistance with feeding.

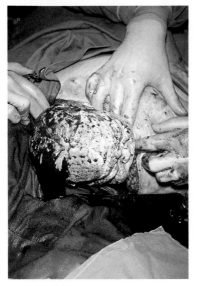

Fig. 196 Head delivered.

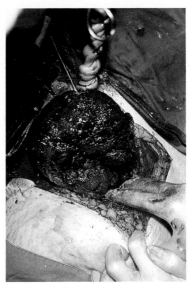

Fig. 197 Delivery of placenta.

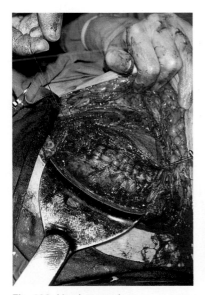

Fig. 198 Uterine repair.

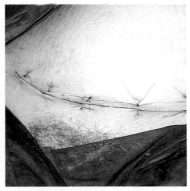

Fig. 199 Skin sutures.

21 | Twins (1)

Incidence

General
Difficult to determine (spontaneous abortion rate is higher, only one twin may be lost). The quoted incidence is 1 in 80 pregnancies although recent reports suggest 1 in 100. Higher-order multiples are much less common: triplets 1 in 80^2, quads 1 in 80^3 (higher incidence with ovulation induction).

Types

Monozygotic (M−Z): results from fertilization of single ovum which divides into two embryos. Rarely share the same sac (1%) and very rarely are conjoined (Fig. 203). No racial or familial predisposition.
Dizygotic (D−Z): results from multiple ovulation and fertilization. Strong familial and racial (Nigerian) predisposition. More frequent with greater maternal age, parity, height and obesity. The M−Z to D−Z ratio is 1:4.

Diagnosis

Large-for-dates, hyperemesis, a raised serum alpha-feto-protein, or early HT. Ultrasound is the best method of diagnosis (Fig. 200). Clinical diagnosis is made by palpating more than two poles or detecting two fetal hearts.

General complications

With the exception of postmaturity, every complication of pregnancy is increased. Accounts for about 10% of perinatal deaths.

Specific complications

Twin-twin transfusion syndrome: due to arteriovenous fistulae through which blood from one fetus drains via the placenta of the other (especially M−Z twins). The donor twin tends to be anaemic and growth-retarded with the recipient twin plethoric and large-for-dates (Fig. 202).

OBSTETRICS

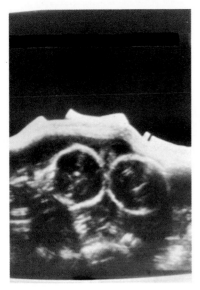

Fig. 200 Diagnosis by ultrasound.

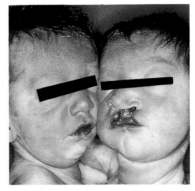

Fig. 201 Risk of congenital anomaly.

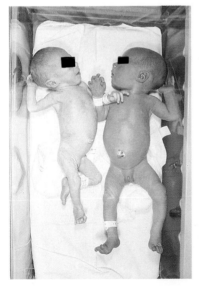

Fig. 202 Discordant growth.

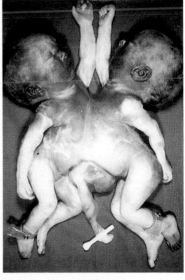

Fig. 203 Conjoined twins.

21 | Twins (2)

Antenatal care

In addition to routine antenatal care:

1. Dietary supplementation of iron and folate.
2. More frequent antenatal checks.
3. Detailed scan at 18 weeks (higher rate of fetal anomalies—Fig. 201).
4. Monthly growth scans thereafter (more often if discordant—Fig. 202).
5. Vigilance for preterm labour.

Labour and delivery

Continuously monitor both fetuses (Fig. 204). Epidural block is the preferred analgesia. Delivery of the first twin is as for a singleton. Delay in delivery of the second twin carries an increased risk of asphyxia. A Syntocinon infusion should be ready (contractions tend to subside after delivery of the first baby). The abdomen is palpated to determine the lie and presentation of the second twin (Fig. 206). A transverse lie is converted to longitudinal either by external version, or by grasping a foot vaginally. With the next contraction the mother recommences pushing and membranes are ruptured. The vagina usually permits easy spontaneous or assisted delivery of the second twin. Two paediatricians and double resuscitation facilities should be available at delivery (Fig. 205). The zygosity can be determined at birth in 80% of twins (sex unlike, or single chorion).

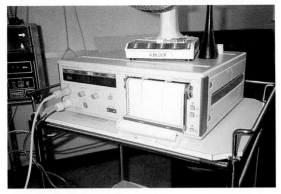

Fig. 204 Double cardiotocography.

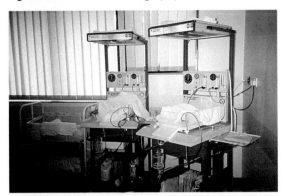

Fig. 205 Double paediatric resources.

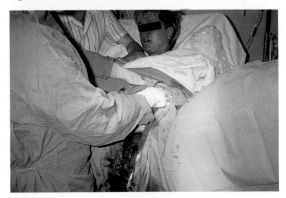

Fig. 206 Palpation of lie of second twin.

22 | Breech Presentation (1)

Incidence

General
Decreases with advancing gestation (25% at 30 weeks and 3% at term).

Aetiology

1. Uterine anomalies, e.g. fibroids, bicornuate uterus.
2. Fetal anomalies, e.g. hydrocephalus, anencephaly.
3. Multiple pregnancy.
4. Placenta praevia.

In most cases no cause is identified.

Types

Frank breech (extended legs) is commonest, then *flexed* and, least commonly, *footling*.

Diagnosis

Antenatal care
Balottable head under costal margin. Confirm with ultrasound.

Management

Check for persistence of breech around 36 weeks. *X-Ray pelvimetry* (Fig. 207). Pelvic diameters of less than 11.0 cm are generally considered inadequate for vaginal delivery. A plain abdominal film (Fig. 208) is also useful for excluding hyperextension of the head (carrying a high risk of spinal cord injury) and gross abnormality. The following should be considered:

1. *External cephalic version* (controversial): the breech is gently displaced upwards and the fetus encouraged to rotate by gentle pressure on either pole. Rh-negative mothers should receive anti-D prophylaxis and the fetus should be monitored afterwards.
2. *Elective Caesarean section:* increasingly used in the past decade, especially in the USA.
3. *Vaginal breech delivery* (see p. 121): if opted for, ultrasound is useful to estimate fetal weight (e.g. by measurement of abdominal circumference) at 38 weeks (Fig. 209), to exclude fetal anomaly and to diagnose a footling presentation.

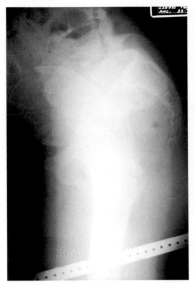

Fig. 207 X-ray pelvimetry.

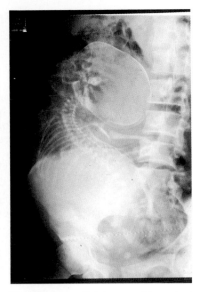

Fig. 208 X-ray fetal normality and attitude.

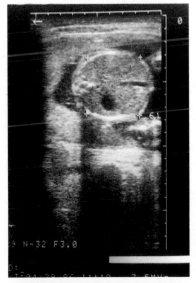

Fig. 209 U/S measurement of fetal abdominal circumference (weight estimation).

Delivery
Relative contra-indications to vaginal delivery:
1. Estimated fetal weight below 1500 g or above 4000 (risk of trauma/asphyxia).
2. Footling presentation (high incidence of cord prolapse).
3. Deflexion attitudes.

Labour

Fetal heart rate monitored continuously. Slow progress and abnormal cardiotocography should be managed by CS, even in the second stage.

Analgesia

Preferably epidural.

Delivery

Pushing is enouraged once the buttocks or feet (Fig. 210) are visible and a generous episiotomy is made with their delivery. Delivery to the umbilicus is by maternal effort alone. If the legs are extended their delivery is assisted by abduction and flexion at the knees (Fig. 211). The arms usually lie across the chest and maternal effort is sufficient to deliver the shoulders. If the arms are extended, a finger is passed over the shoulder to the antecubital fossa which is flexed and the arm brought down (Fig. 212). The fetus is either allowed to hang or delivered along the attendant's arm until the hairline is visible. Delivery of the head is controlled by laying the trunk astride an arm with a finger in the mouth and the other hand on the occiput (Mauriceau Smellie Veit manoeuvre), or by applying forceps after lifting the feet (Fig. 213).

Complications

Asphyxia: cord compression or entrapment of head in incompletely dilated cervix.
Trauma: e.g. abdominal viscera, spinal cord, brachial plexus.

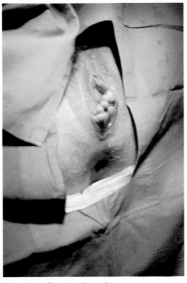

Fig. 210 Feet at introitus.

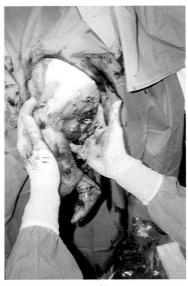

Fig. 211 Delivery of legs.

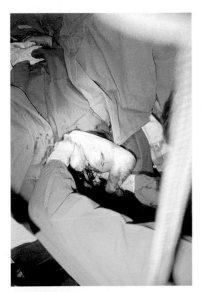

Fig. 212 Delivery of arms.

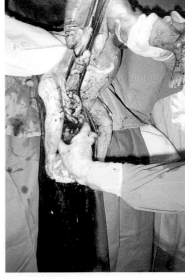

Fig. 213 Delivery of head (forceps).

Definition

Cephalhaematoma (Fig. 214)
Fluctuant mass loosely attached under the periosteum of cranial bones (commonly parietal) and not crossing the suture lines.

Incidence

0.5−2.5% of vaginal deliveries.

Aetiology

May follow spontaneous delivery but more commonly follows forceps or ventouse (3%).

Course

May contribute to anaemia and jaundice. Usually resolves spontaneously over several weeks. Rarely calcification or infection occur.

Ventouse extraction
Scalp echymoses and artificial caput (chignon) always occur (Fig. 215). Chignon diminishes markedly in the first hour following delivery. Scalp abrasions (8%) take longer to resolve and necrosis is rare.

Forceps
Facial pressure marks (Fig. 216) are very common and disappear within hours. Abrasions may take some days to heal but rarely leave scars.

Facial palsy (Fig. 217).
Presents as asymmetry of the face on crying.

Incidence

About 0.25% of births.

Aetiology

Compression of the facial nerve distal to the stylomastoid foramen during labour or delivery. More common following forceps but can follow normal delivery due to pressure on a maternal bony prominence or the fetus's own shoulder.

Management

Protect the eye which cannot be closed (lower motor neurone lesion).

Course

Most cases resolve within days.

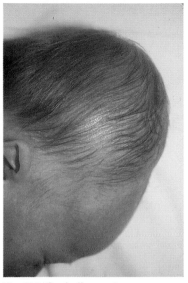

Fig. 214 Cephalhaematoma.

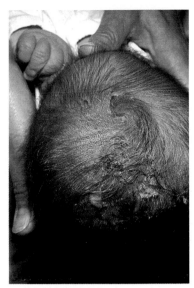

Fig. 215 Ventouse.

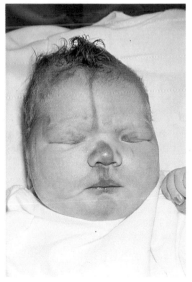

Fig. 216 Forceps mark.

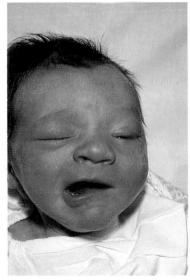

Fig. 217 Facial palsy.

Vaginal breech delivery predisposes to certain types of injury including spinal cord lesions, peripheral nerve palsies, fractures of long bones and intracranial bleeding. Bruising of the genitalia (Fig. 218) is very common and resolves without long-term sequele, although this is less certain in males.

Types

Brachial plexus injuries
1. *Erb's palsy* (97%) (lesion of C5, 6): internal rotation of arm with extension and adduction of hand; rarely phrenic nerve palsy (Fig. 219).
2. *Klumpke's palsy* (3%) (Lesion of C8, T1): weakness of hand, rarely with Horner's syndrome.

Aetiology

Traction on bracheal plexus during delivery. More common after shoulder dystocia.

Prognosis

80% recover completely in 3–6 months. Occasionally there is severe permanent deficit resulting in a functionless short limb.

Aetiology

Tentorial tear (Fig. 220)
Hypoxia renders the brain oedematous and its supporting membranes rigid and prone to damage. Excessive moulding, prematurity, breech and forceps delivery are further predisposing factors.

Course

The infant is usually flaccid, pale and difficult to resuscitate at birth. Survivors have high incidence of neurological sequelae.

Injuries to intra-abdominal viscera
Tearing of the liver (Fig. 221) or spleen may follow breech delivery and is avoided by minimizing handling. Intraperitoneal haemorrhage results in shock and anaemia, and sometimes blood in the scrotum. Urgent laporotomy may be necessary.

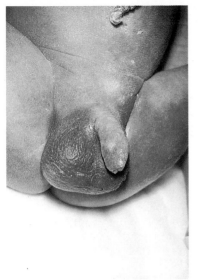

Fig. 218 Bruised genitalia.

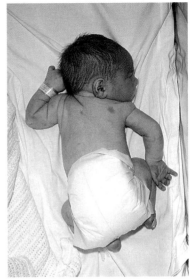

Fig. 219 Erb's palsy.

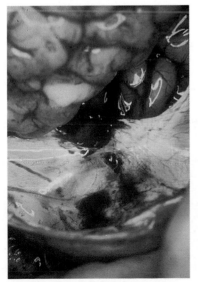

Fig. 220 Tentorial tear.

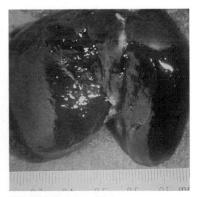

Fig. 221 Ruptured liver.

Injuries associated with fetal monitoring
A scalp abscess at the site of electrode application occurs in 0.5–5%. These usually resolve spontaneously with a small minority requiring surgical drainage and antibiotics. Removal of a piece of scalp (Fig. 222) occurred when the electrode was pulled off at delivery. Fortunately, plastic surgical repair gave a good result (Fig. 223).

Subconjunctival haemorrhages (Fig. 224)
These may be found following vaginal birth in both infant and mother (Fig. 231, p. 131). They resolve spontaneously and do not require any special management.

Injuries associated with Caesarean section
All of the injuries mentioned in association with vaginal delivery have also been reported after Caesarean section. Although widely regarded as a safer mode of delivery for the infant, delivery by this route can occasionally be as difficult and traumatic as a vaginal delivery. Laceration of the fetus is only likely to occur at Caesarean section and often involves the face (Fig. 225). This may result in an unsightly scar and may need treatment in the form of plastic surgery.

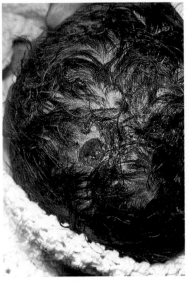

Fig. 222 Avulsion of scalp skin by scalp electrode.

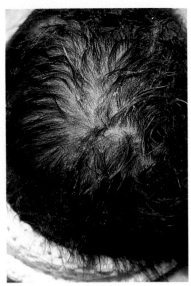

Fig. 223 Sutured scalp.

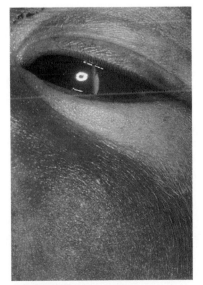

Fig. 224 Subconjunctival haemorrhage.

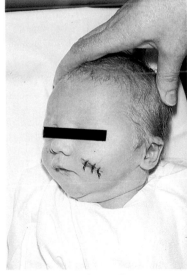

Fig. 225 Laceration at Caesarean section.

| # The Puerperium (1)

Definition

The interval following labour taken to return to the normal non-pregnant state. Conventionally taken as 6 weeks, although most anatomical changes are complete within 2 weeks. In the UK it is a statutory requirement for mothers to be seen daily for 10–14 days by a midwife who routinely checks blood pressure, temperature, scars, lochia, breasts and involution of the uterus (Fig. 226), and also checks that the infant is well and advises on feeding difficulties.

Maternal complications

Puerperal sepsis: defined as a temperature of 38°C or more within 14 days of delivery. The usual causes are included in the following complications.

Perineum: perineal pain is extremely common following vaginal delivery and results from bruising (Fig. 227), oedema (Fig. 228) and infection. Analgesia, frequent bathing and removal of any tight sutures provide symtomatic relief. In more severe cases a course of perineal ultrasound may be beneficial.

Vagina: vaginal haematomas (Fig. 229) are less common. Presentation is with increasingly severe pain in the rectum, usually within 6 hours of delivery. The pain is often refractory to opiate analgesia, and the haematoma is palpable on vaginal or rectal examination. Management is by surgical evacuation of the clot, haemostasis and resuturing of the vagina and perineum. The amount of blood contained may be sufficient to make the patient anaemic.

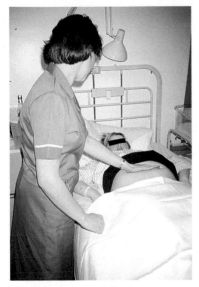

Fig. 226 Post-natal check.

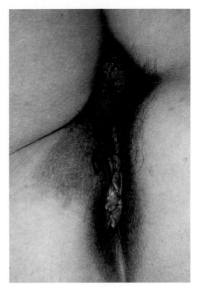

Fig. 227 Perineal bruising.

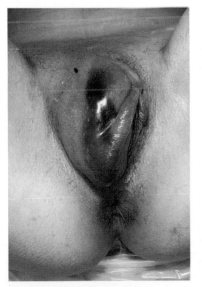

Fig. 228 Perineal oedema.

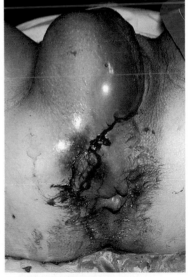

Fig. 229 Vaginal haematoma.

| # The Puerperium (2)

Maternal complications (contd)

Haemorrhoids: a common complaint in pregnancy due to caval compression. They are prone to thrombosis and prolapse at delivery resulting in painful oedematous haemorrhoids (Fig. 230), a major source of puerperal discomfort. Management is by replacement of prolapsed haemorrhoids, analgesia (systemic and topical) and measures to prevent constipation.

Eyes: subconjunctival haemorrhages (Fig. 231) may result from maternal expulsive efforts during the second stage. They are asymptomatic and resolve spontaneously.

Wound infection or haematoma (Fig. 232): follows in 10% of Caesarean sections. They delay healing and when associated with a vertical incision, occasionally give rise to wound dehiscence (rare with transverse incision). Chest infection, thrombo-embolism, ileus, urinary tract infection and anaemia are also more common than following vaginal delivery.

Uterus. Infection (endometritis) is usually at the placental site and presents with pyrexia, abdominal discomfort and vaginal bleeding. Treatment is with antibiotics and analgesia. Uterine rupture (Fig. 233) is fortunately rare, arising in about 1 in 2000 deliveries. Most ruptures occur during labour. In primigravidae rupture only occurs in association with previous uterine surgery, uterine manipulation or instrumental delivery. Multigravidae are more at risk, most ruptures occurring in a previous CS scar, especially vertical (classical) scars.

OBSTETRICS

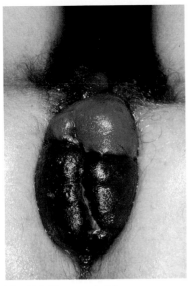

Fig. 230 Haemorrhoids.

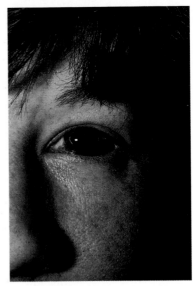

Fig. 231 Subconjunctival hemorrhages.

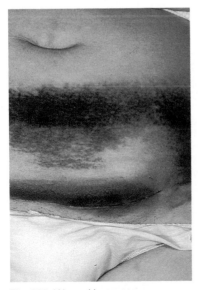

Fig. 232 Wound haematoma.

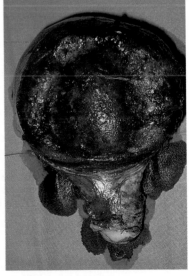

Fig. 233 Ruptured uterus.

Maternal complications (contd)

Breast: engorgement normally occurs on days 2 to 4. Mastitis (Fig. 234) is relatively common and starts with reddening and tenderness progressing to an oedematous induration with fever and malaise.

Aetiology

Staphylococci or streptococci, usually introduced by the baby during suckling, particularly on a cracked nipple, often with stasis of milk in a breast lobule or a blocked duct.

Management

Antibiotics (flucloxacillin), analgesics and regular emptying of the breast (infection is not a contra-indication to continuing breast feeding). Neglected mastitis will progress to abscess formation requiring surgical drainage.

Suppression

For mothers not wishing to breast feed, firm support, avoidance of suckling and analgesia are usually sufficient. In circumstances where breast feeding is contra-indicated (e.g. following certain types of breast surgery, or in mothers who have experienced perinatal death), pharmacological suppression with bromocriptine (Fig. 235) may be indicated. Oestrogens are contra-indicated because of the risk of thrombo-embolism.
Pituitary: postpartum necrosis of the anterior pituitary (Fig. 236) giving rise to Sheehan's syndrome results from severe postpartum haemorrhage and shock. It is avoided by prompt management of haemorrhage, and now rarely occurs. The earliest presenting symptom is failure of lactation followed by amenorrhoea. Lifetime replacement of pituitary trophic hormones or those of their target organs is necessary.

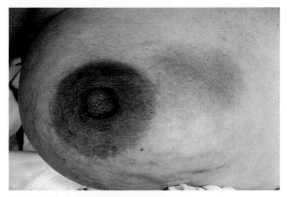

Fig. 234 Breast infection/mastitis.

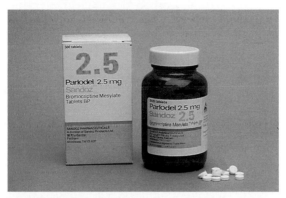

Fig. 235 Bromocriptine.

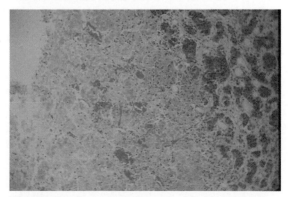

Fig. 236 Histology of pituitary gland in Sheehan's syndrome.

Following pregnancy sexual activity may be resumed as soon as it is comfortable to do so, usually after a couple of weeks, by which time most anatomical changes of pregnancy have regressed. The endocrine changes take longer, and return to fertility is variable and may be delayed for months by lactation. Non-lactating mothers may ovulate within 4 weeks of delivery and return of menstruation occurs on average at 58 days. It is extremely rare for fully breast feeding women to ovulate or menstruate prior to 10 weeks. Breast feeding alone, however, is not a reliable contraceptive method.

Hormonal methods
It is safe to use these in the puerperium bearing in mind the usual contra-indications to use of oestrogen-containing preparations (history of prior thrombo-embolism, cerebrovascular accident or hypertension).

Types

Combined oestrogen/progestogen pills (Fig. 237): taken cyclically, they suppress gonadotrophins and should be started within 3 weeks of delivery if not breast feeding, or when lactation ceases as they may suppress milk production. Blood pressure and weight are checked regularly and cervical cytology every 3 years.
Progestogen-only formulations: no serious side effects, but they can cause menstrual irregularity. Oral preparations (Fig. 238) must be taken daily starting the second week after delivery. Alternatively, they can be given by deep intramuscular injection (Fig. 239) lasting about 3 months.

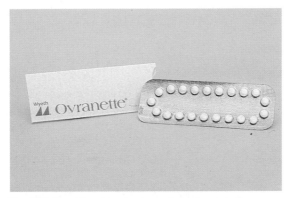

Fig. 237 Combined oestrogen-progestogen pill.

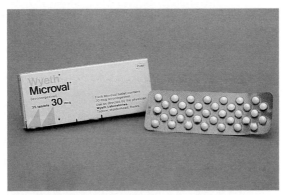

Fig. 238 Progestogen-only pill.

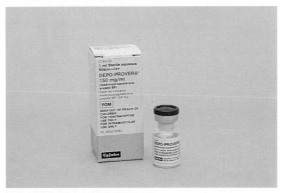

Fig. 239 Depot progestogen.

Intra-uterine devices

Insertion can be undertaken at any time in the puerperium. In general, however, expulsion rates are higher when insertion is earlier and thus, this is usually deferred until 6 weeks.

Types

There are many varieties but they fall into two types: inert devices and those containing copper. Inert devices (Fig. 240) can be left in situ for many years but have more side effects than do the smaller, copper-containing devices (Fig. 241). The latter also have lower pregnancy rates but need to be changed every 2–3 years.

Complications

1. Pelvic pain, menorrhagia and intermenstrual bleeding are common.
2. Pelvic inflammatory disease is more common than with other methods of contraception.
3. Uterine perforation. This probably occurs during insertion but usually only becomes apparent when the threads cannot be located subsequently. The location of the coil can be ascertained with ultrasound (Fig. 242) and surgical intervention may be necessary for removal.
4. The rate of ectopic pregnancy is higher than with other methods, except possibly hormonal regimens containing only progestogen.
5. Pregnancy. In the event of failure the spontaneous abortion rate is high.

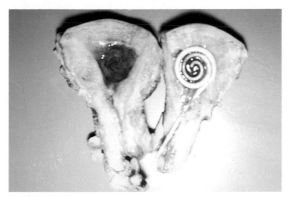

Fig. 240 A plastic IUCD in sectioned uterus.

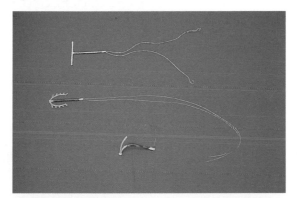

Fig. 241 Copper devices.

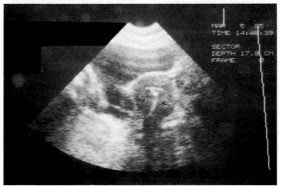

Fig. 242 IUCD in situ on ultrasound.

25 | Contraception (3)

Barrier contraception
Unlike other methods, these offer some
protection against sexually transmited diseases;
however, they have a slightly higher failure rate
and additional use of spermicides is advisable as
it improves their efficacy.

Types | *Diaphragm* (Fig. 243): fits behind the cervix,
covers it and is tucked up behind the symphysis
pubis. The correct size needs to be assessed
(often different after childbirth), and the patient
taught to fit and check the diaphragm herself. It
should be left in situ for several hours after
intercourse.
Cervical cap: just covers the cervix and is similar,
in principle, to the diaphragm.
Condom/sheath (Fig. 244): a thin, rubber penile
sheath with a reservoir to collect ejaculate.

Natural family planning
This requires self-recognition of ovulation by
examination of cervical mucus and basal
temperature. The changes of the puerperium and
influence of lactation make such recognition
difficult.

Sterilization
Only appropriate for those desiring permanent
contraception. Tubal ligation or diathermy may
be undertaken at the time of Caesarean section or
in the early puerperium (by mini-laparotomy);
however, the thickness and vascularity of the
tubes at this time results in a higher failure rate.
Delaying the procedure until after the puerperium
enables laparoscopic sterilization at which a small
portion of tube is occluded by application of a
silastic ring or clip (Fig. 245).

OBSTETRICS

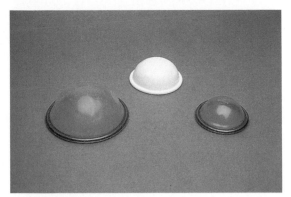

Fig. 243 Diaphragm.

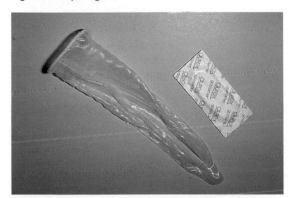

Fig. 244 Sheath.

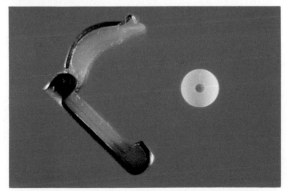

Fig. 245 Filshie clip and Falop ring for sterilization.

Index